Asymmetrical Conversations

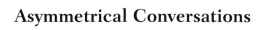

Asymmetrical Conversations

Contestations, Circumventions, and the Blurring of Therapeutic Boundaries

Edited by
Harish Naraindas, Johannes Quack,
and William S. Sax

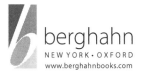

berghahn
NEW YORK · OXFORD
www.berghahnbooks.com

First published in 2014 by
Berghahn Books
www.berghahnbooks.com

Library of Congress Cataloging-in-Publication Data
Asymmetrical conversations : contestations, circumventions, and the blurring
of therapeutic boundaries / edited by Harish Naraindas, Johannes Quack, and
William S. Sax.
    p. ; cm. — (Epistemologies of healing ; volume 14)
    Includes bibliographical references and index.
    ISBN 978-1-78238-308-6 (hbk. : alk. paper) — ISBN 978-1-78238-309-3
ebook)
    I. Naraindas, Harish, editor of compilation.   II. Quack, Johannes, editor
of compilation.   III. Sax, William Sturman, 1957– editor of compilation.
IV. Series: Epistemologies of healing ; v. 14.
[DNLM: 1. Mind-Body Relations, Metaphysical.   2. Medicine, Ayurvedic.
3. Spiritual Therapies. WB 880]
    RZ401
    615.5—dc23   2013033636

British Library Cataloguing in Publication Data
A catalogue record for this book is available from the British Library

Printed on acid-free paper

ISBN: 978-1-78238-308-6 hardback
ISBN: 978-1-78238-309-3 ebook

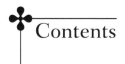

Contents

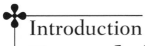

Introduction
Entangled Epistemes

Harish Naraindas, Johannes Quack,
and William S. Sax

Natural, Contingent, and Plausible Worlds

Most people's understandings of the body, their models of health and disease, their ideas about appropriate modes of treatment, and their assumptions about the right places to get such treatment seem quite natural to them. They regard such ideas as rational and scientific (though often imperfect) responses to disease, as divinely sanctioned paradigms for understanding illness and acting upon it, or simply as "the way things are," and as such, they rarely question them. But the social sciences and especially the medical humanities—disciplines like medical anthropology, history of medicine, and cultural psychiatry—teach us that such ideas are not as "natural" as they might seem. Rather, they change over time and according to political and economic conditions, and are related to factors like "caste," "class," "race," and "gender." In short, they are socioculturally shaped and historically contingent.

But if such ideas are contingent, how is it that they come to be regarded as natural and plausible? The answer has partly to do with their internal coherence and plausibility in a wider cultural and historical context. Somehow or other they must be consistent with other ideas: about the world and human beings' place in it, about the connection between morality and disease, about the proper relationship between healers and patients, and about a host of other matters. Much work in the medical humanities has focused on the "fit" between health-related ideas and the wider cosmologies and social systems in which they are embedded. This is particularly evident in

1

discussions of the relationships between healers (including medical doctors) and patients. For quite a long time, writers in the medical humanities assumed that "explanatory models of illness" were usually shared between healers and patients, and that this common ground of understanding was of crucial importance for effective therapy. This assumption has recently been challenged (for an overview see Quack 2013). But that is not the whole story, and in fact it may not even be the right story. In recent decades, scholars have increasingly argued that in addition to forms of knowledge (whether shared or unshared), specific, health-related *practices* are also of great importance for understanding how therapy unfolds, whether or not it works, etc.

The main catalyst for this practical turn was Pierre Bourdieu, who convincingly argued that practices are neither secondary nor opposed to beliefs, nor do they arise directly out of beliefs, but rather that practices and beliefs are mutually constitutive. It is not simply that we kneel in church because we believe ourselves to be subordinate to God: equally importantly, the practice of kneeling (for example by children before they even form coherent beliefs about their relationship to God) produces bodily dispositions that might result in the generation of subordinate believers. In the realm of health -seeking, it is not simply that we defer to the greater wisdom of the physician out of intellectual conviction: of equal importance is the fact that the practices associated with doctors' offices and hospitals (registering at the front desk, taking a seat in the waiting room until one is summoned, being required to shed normal dress and don certain kinds of depersonalizing clothing in the hospital, etc.) produce an attitude of deference and passivity.

In other words, we are socialized into systems of belief by a series of concrete bodily acts and other complex practices that make the world a naturalized and taken-for-granted entity where things are done in such and such a way. And these systems of belief and practice are historical artifacts that are co-constituted as regimes of truth and of power. Nevertheless, some scholars persist in explaining people's health care behavior exclusively in terms of explicitly held beliefs. We do not deny that socializations into bodily dispositions are often accompanied by appropriate verbal expressions and shaped by larger cosmologies, which can be elaborated to a greater or lesser degree. But the illness models people produce are also embedded in a set of bodily dispositions, which were theorized by Mauss (1935), Elias (1939), and Bourdieu (1998) in different yet related ways as "habitus." This term has become central to the social sciences, and bears a great deal of theoretical weight, not least because it is differently theorized by different authors. For our purposes, what is important about the notion of "habitus" is that it refers to personal dispositions that are not so much the products of reflective thought as of socialization; bodily and behavioral expressions of one's position in social space. Habitus is important for this volume because it points to the fact that what is called "health-seeking behavior" is not simply a matter of rational choice.

Institutions, Practices, and Beliefs

Such observations are now common in the literature. But what is often underemphasized is how such beliefs and practices, or modes of thought and codes of conduct, relate to formal institutions: not just the hospitals mentioned above, but also, for example, spaces where the body is cultivated (fitness centers, beauty parlors, athletic venues); where illness is diagnosed (clinics, diviners' huts, X-ray rooms); or where healing takes place (operating theaters, churches, physiotherapy centers).[1] Furthermore, such ideas and practices are produced and reinforced in familial, educational, and professional contexts where people learn about how to properly dress and comport themselves, about what they should and should not eat, and how they should treat other people's bodies; as well as in institutionalized contexts (life-cycle rituals, sporting events, parades and marches, classrooms, offices, factory floors, etc.), where bodies are evaluated, marked, and defined as healthy or ill, normal or pathological. It is here that the works of Michel Foucault and Georges Canguilhem are seminal. Canguilhem (1978) showed how medical ideas about "the normal," and medical processes of normalization, were inextricably bound up with the Industrial Revolution and the introduction of "norms" in sanitary practices, architecture, engineering, etc., in fact, with the whole edifice of a rising industrial society and a social class—the bourgeoisie—that required the norm and the normal as regulatory mechanisms to mark, compare, evaluate, judge, confine, treat, discipline, exclude, include, produce, promote, and punish.

3

In the realm of medicine this is best exemplified by the coming into being of the teaching hospital, or the "birth of the clinic" (Foucault 1973), where practice in the double sense of pedagogy and clinical practice, or the creation and transmission of knowledge, was housed in a particular institution, engendering new relationships between the subject and object of knowledge, between doctor and patient, and between modes of philanthropy, economic assistance, and the very constitution of knowledge. This led to an ontological and epistemological recasting of "health" and "disease," which were now apprehended in terms of the Normal and the Pathological (Foucault 1973), thus testifying to a new relationship among knowledge, institution, and practice.

The teaching hospital exemplifies this coming together of the cognitive, the practical, and the normative, and this is consistent with one of our fundamental assumptions: that in order to understand the complex relations among concepts of body and mind, notions of health and disease, patterns of treatment-seeking, and modes of therapy, it is important to look at the relationships among the triad of ideas, practices, and the institutions in which they are manifest. We take very seriously the idea that health-related beliefs and practices are largely determined by such relationships, and that they acquire plausibility, stability, and "taken-for-grantedness" when ideas, practices, and institutions reinforce each other. This is another example of the "looping effect" (Hacking 1999; Kirmayer and Sartorius 2007), where new forms of knowledge about human beings produce new kinds of experts, who classify and treat people according to their expert knowledge, sometimes producing what Hacking has called new "human kinds," the existence of which reinforces and transforms the forms of knowledge and practices upon which their identification as "kinds" initially depended. Prominent examples in the literature include trauma (Young 1995), multiple personality disorder, and models of human development (Hacking 1995), all of which have altered our notions of what it means to be human.

While none of the authors in this volume goes so far as to suggest that he or she is describing the creation of a new "human kind," there is nevertheless something similar happening, since what is at stake in most cases is the competition between alternative ontologies of the body, with their associated epistemologies of health, disease, and therapy. The crucial point is that this competition is not simply a matter of ideas, but rather a question of the mutual reinforcement of ideas, institutions, and practices. Such "looping" involves iteration and reiteration, but not merely on a linguistic or a conceptual level. Rather, ideas, practices, and institutions reinforce each other. The more inclusive such loops are—that is, the more they include other realms like politics, religion, or economics—the more powerful and stable they are, and the more "natural" they seem. And with this process of naturalization, they become all the more difficult to circumvent. In the United States, for example, ideas about individual ownership of, and responsibility for, the body are reinforced by the institutions and ideology of market capitalism, by the ethic of "rugged individualism," by a privatized medical system, and by the commercialization of "spiritual" therapies. In rural India, by contrast, ideas about permeable and transacting bodies, and the embedding of the individual within the family, are reinforced by collective decision making in the hospital as well as at the healer's shrine.

But although cultural styles and their looping effects are important for stabilizing and naturalizing the habitus, the reality today is that institutions and ideologies of market capitalism and biomedicine intrude deeply into all the health systems in our globalized world. This has led some to question the importance of cultural difference in the production of illness (Farmer 2003); and others to argue that global forms of health care always produce particular local adaptations (cf. Robertson 1995). Indeed, most of the articles in this volume wrestle with precisely this tension between the global and the local, and their particular negotiated settlements. What happens, for example, when institutionalized psychiatry under state auspices physically intrudes into a healing shrine (Basu, this volume), or when traditional nosologies are compelled to redefine themselves in biomedical terms (Naraindas, 2006)? How can Indians visit a psychiatric ward one day, and on the next day participate in ritual practices involving "possession" (Quack this volume)? How do traditional healers in Kerala combine exorcism with modern Ayurvedic medicines (Sax and Bhaskar, this volume)?

These self-reinforcing loops among institutions, practices, and concepts are, however, neither innocent nor symmetrical. On the contrary, they are shaped by many (often invisible) underlying asymmetries. There is a body of established scholarship discussing how the realm of health and well-being is marked by one overwhelming asymmetry: the scientific, economic, and institutional domination of biomedicine (also called "modern medicine"; "cosmopolitan medicine"; "allopathy," in India; and *Schulmedizin*, in Germany). It is one of the most successful Western exports ever, subduing or annexing other medical approaches. Biomedicine has penetrated nearly every corner of the globe, so that most adults living in the twenty-first century know what doctors are and the "right" way to consult them, what injections are and how one makes use of them, what hospitals are and why one visits them. Biomedicine is ideologically, scientifically, financially, and politically dominant nearly everywhere, and that is why a further thread connecting the articles in this volume is the asymmetry between it and other forms of healing. Our recognition of this fact is, however, coupled with our uneasiness about the associated oppositions of modern versus traditional, scientific versus religious, Western versus Eastern, biomedicine versus indigenous medicine, body versus mind, individual versus dividual, and curing versus healing. These oppositions, which are rough homologues of one another, with a similar asymmetrical structure privileging the first term, seem to structure the pedagogy and practice of contemporary modes of healing, not just in India or South Asia, but worldwide. But we hope that the chapters in this volume will succeed in questioning their "naturalness" or inevitability by showing that they, too, are not simply ideas, but also structures created by institutions and practices in relation to ideas, and therefore necessarily implicated in power, politics, and resistance.

Circumventing Ideologies

It often transpires that people seek to bypass, circumvent, or even transcend the dominant ideologies of their cultures as these are manifested in the typical institutions of health care: contemporary Asians strive to be "modern individualists"; Westerners want to be holistic and in touch with "nature." Alternative therapies thrive: Ayurveda and yoga in Europe, Reiki and Pranik Healing in South Asia. Many people feel that their health systems objectify them, paying attention only to their physical illnesses, and they seek therapies offering some kind of spiritual transcendence. Or they feel that their legitimate physical complaints are not being adequately addressed, and prefer a purely somatic diagnosis, or a prescription for strong medication.

In these and other ways, people can and do ignore, circumvent, and even resist dominant cultural paradigms of health, illness, and care, as illustrated by the chapters in this volume: sometimes by introducing new modes of therapy (Warrier), at other times by continuing their preferred therapies in the face of opposition by the state or the medical establishment (Basu), by "converting" patients to minority therapies (Sax and Bhaskar), by choosing an alternative therapy even when it is frowned upon by family and friends (Naraindas), and sometimes by making use of all available therapeutic options at once (Quack). One possibility, explored by Sax and Bhaskar, is that the oppositions Modern/Traditional, West/East, etc., are more ideological than real; that is, that they reflect medical or scholarly paradigms that are belied by practice. More generally, attempts to circumvent dominant ideologies of health normally take place in the context of systems that are marked by numerous asymmetries: for example between healers and sufferers, competing medical systems, or public and private providers. A healing system that has the support of the state apparatus with its regulatory functions has distinct advantages over one that does not: the latter can hardly generate the comprehensive social-economic-political "loops" of the former, and the inability to do so is both a cause and consequence of its weaker position. Warrier shows, however, that Ayurveda was able to capitalize on the creative freedom afforded by its marginal position as it emerged in the U.K., partly by embracing and partly by resisting the government's regulatory initiatives, thereby holding its formal institutional aspects and its informal networks in creative tension with each other. Against this background we do not postulate an easygoing, "live-and-let-live" form of medical pluralism where people unproblematically choose among alternative forms of therapy, sometimes using more than one at the same time; rather, we want to stress the implicit asymmetries that shape health-seeking behavior and the positioning of medical systems against one another, as well as the occasional and deliberate rejection of dominant models of regulation and institutionalization in favor of alternative ones. This is not always entirely successful: the intention or desire to bypass, circumvent, or transcend the "dispositions" into which one has been socialized, or the dominant paradigms in one's social field, may not succeed at all, or it may succeed only partially, resulting in a mangling of practices—since institutional constraints, at times including

7

legal ones, often make it impossible to avoid the dominant paradigm. In such cases people are compelled to negotiate, and may shuttle between practices and systems, create protocols and practices, or devise nosological categories and therapeutic strategies that fulfill the techno-legal requirements of the institutions that they are seeking to bypass, while still allowing them to pursue (sometimes covertly) their therapies of choice (Basu, Naraindas, and Warrier, this volume). In the bargain, and through these ontological enactments—that is, through their beings and bodies and not merely with their heads—those seeking health may produce new objects, therapies, and institutional forms by a continuous conversation that is forever in the making.

South Asia as an Exemplary Epistemological Cauldron

What distinguishes this volume from the existing body of scholarship on medicine in South Asia? First of all, it establishes new ways of focusing on the *experiential* trajectories or consequences for patients choosing a particular therapy in the shadow of overarching asymmetries, thus drawing most of its evidence from ethnographic research. Second, it combines studies of somatic and mental "pathologies," and of textual as well as oral traditions. Finally and most importantly, it brings *practices* (including linguistic practices), *institutions, and ideas* together in a single overarching argument. Through a disciplinary division of labor, we have attempted to bring together this triad, not by looking at the numerous paths to Asian Medical Knowledge through their "ideational practices" (Leslie 1976; Leslie and Young 1992), nor by looking at the several avatars of the dominant South Asian system, namely Ayurveda, in its diasporic or global form (Reddy 2002, 2004; Wujastyck and Smith 2008), nor by focusing on the pharmaceuticalization, industrialization, and commercialization of Ayurveda and other South Asian medical traditions (Bode 2008; Banerjee 2009). We focus neither on somatic health nor mental health exclusively (Ecks 2005; Ecks and Basu 2009; Halliburton 2009; Sébastia 2009). This collection is not intended as a history of one or several "systems" of South Asian Medicine and their reconfigurations under colonial dispensation (Attewell 2007), or of Western medical practices in colonial India (Ernst 1991). It is not an attempt to condense the several styles of their contemporary practice in India under a single label (Langford 2002), thereby distinguishing them from biomedicine; nor do we seek to use medicine as a prism to talk about nationalism or the making of regional, religious, and ethnic identities (Sivaramakrishnan 2006).

Although we find these studies useful and often inspiring, we focus on a different, but central problematic: the dualism of mind and body, and how this plays itself out in institutions, practices, and ideas. We argue that because biomedicine is so overwhelmingly dominant throughout the world, the many forms of "alternative" medicine are compelled to position themselves in relation to this basic, structuring dualism: either by reiterating it (representing themselves as exclusively "spiritual"), redefining it (discovering it in their own pasts), or challenging it (representing themselves as "holistic"). It is not unusual for a "medical system" to follow all of these paths, via its several manifestations: Ayurveda tends to represent itself globally as "holistic and green" (Zimmermann 1992) and in Europe as "spiritual" (Warrier, this volume), while in India it is busy inventing the subdiscipline of Ayurvedic psychiatry as a special science of mind (Halliburton 2009; Lang and Jansen 2013). Overall, the mind/body dualism separates not only somatic from mental pathology, but also the diseases of doctors from the illnesses of patients, and the "learned traditions" from the "vernacular practices," where the former (in their "modern" forms) deal primarily with medical problems while the latter consist primarily of religious beliefs and practices often described as "magic" and "superstition." Vernacular traditions must therefore either own the distinction, and be content with their definition as "nonmodern" and "nonscientific," or they must work creatively with the dichotomy so as to obtain a higher place in the global hierarchy of knowledge. Seen through this prism, South Asia is an arena in which these asymmetrical relations play themselves out to the full, presumably because so many forms of "textual/learned" traditions and "oral/vernacular" practices still coexist, making it an exemplary epistemological cauldron. Although the South Asian setting is important, this collection of chapters is focused rather on a particular argument (along with several subsidiary ones), attempting to show how an overarching dualism produces several types of asymmetrical conversations between the marginalized and the mainstream, what each of these conversations entail, how protagonists equivocate and struggle, and what the consequences and experiences of this "cooking" in the South Asian cauldron are.

Entailments and Equivocations

Against such a backdrop this volume examines two things. First, what kind of practices do certain institutions "ask for" or entail? The internal spaces of health-related institutions call forth particular responses: a certain kind of behavior is called for by the simple act of entering a hospital rather than a health resort, or a healing shrine rather than a mental institution. What are the differences between the way people speak and act when they seek treatment in a hospital, as opposed to a temple? What kind of pressure is exercised by such institutions on patients and practitioners? What difficulties and hurdles are faced by those wishing to circumvent dominant medical systems? Our focus on how institutions require certain kinds of behavior also shows how they reinforce ideas and practices relating to health, illness, and therapy.

Second, what happens when people are either unwilling or unable to "comply" with the practices appropriate to or necessary for the therapeutic processes in a given institution? How do such people equivocate, circumvent, resist, transcend, or negotiate the ideological and institutional constraints that are dominant in their particular cultural and historical contexts? We trace, on the one hand, the constraints of local (and sometimes global) ideologies and institutions, and how people circumvent or resist them; on the other hand we examine what Latour (1993) would call the "purifying" activities of professional organizations, government bureaucrats, lawyers, and others who try to keep such rules in place. In other words, what transpires between these institutional constraints on the one hand and attempts to get around them on the other?

It is important to notice that recourse to alternative therapies is only possible when such alternatives are at hand. Their range and number vary, from the creative individual in a culturally conservative context who invents a new healing ritual, or discovers a new medicinal herb, to the plethora of alternatives available in a Southeast Asian market or a modern industrial city. And in practice, the availability of alternative therapies is also constrained by ideologies, economics, and issues of access, as well as by institutions. Hospitals, insurance companies, shrines, families: each generate their own moral, religious, economic, cognitive, and bodily demands, normative orders that are explicitly articulated or constitute unarticulated background conditions, so that the costs of "resisting," "circumventing," or simply being an Other to a dominant healing system can be considerable, in some cases even life-threatening (Naraindas, this volume). It is thus evident that what the chapters here grapple with are *conversations* of various kinds under the sign of asymmetry.

Asymmetrical Conversations

The opening chapter by Laurence Kirmayer reviews the history of the mind/body dualism and its continuing persistence in the Western tradition. It ranges over a host of topics in its review of the many meanings and usages of "imagination." Kirmayer starts with an understanding of imagination as a central ability of the mind, and discusses the roots of the mind/body dualism in ancient Greece. From there he moves to imagination's role in the medicine of the early Renaissance, for example in the medical approach of Paracelsus as well as the emergence of rationalism and scientific empiricism with its rejection of "metaphorical imagination." Here a moment was missed when, in an attempt to debunk mesmerism in the nineteenth century, the effects of hypnosis were seen as resulting from the gullibility and credulity of some minds that, due to personal frailties and an "overheated imagination," were vulnerable to suggestion. According to the Royal Commission constituted to evaluate mesmerism, minds open to suggestion were deficient. The commission failed to see that all minds, given the right conditions, are open to suggestion, a recognition that would have paved the way for the imagination to be rightfully part of a therapeutic and/or diagnostic process. This can be understood as a particular kind of mistrust of the mind in post-Enlightenment Europe. Kirmayer reviews the European history of the imagination and the mind, and shows that the gap wrought by this mistrust is partly filled by what are today called CAMs, that is, Complementary and Alternative Medicines. Hence, it is none too surprising that many if not all of them have been christened "mind-body medicine."

Kirmayer makes it clear that CAMs are marked by a variety of epistemologies and ontologies. In the contemporary, globalized marketplace, not only are claims on their behalf often overstated, but most such systems have been disembedded from their original traditions and are offered under the general rubric of "holistic medicine," often as gentle alternatives to biomedicine (cf. Zimmermann 1992), which in turn is seen as impersonal, fragmented, and toxic. Given this rhetorical construction of CAMs, it is not surprising that in the contemporary medical medley, the choice of a particular therapy on the part of a patient, or practitioner, is often the sign of solidarity with others sharing similar views, or identification with a particular aesthetics or stance that this alternative therapy is seen to represent.

Kirmayer concludes by suggesting that the way out of this apparently dead end, which is premised on the persistence of mind/body dualism, is to give both mind and body full play in both prognosis and therapy. In a perceptive section he dwells on this possibility within the dominant tradition and its subdiscipline of psychosomatic medicine, which attempts to bridge the gap. But the dualism is so strong that its erasure becomes very difficult indeed.

The next chapter, by Johannes Quack, compares two therapeutic institutions where mind and body are quite differently at play in prognosis and therapy: on the one hand, possession experiences at the *Balaji* healing temple, and on the other a psychiatric out-patient department (OPD) in India. Quack argues that the "shrine environment" of *Balaji* at Mehndipur induces possession in some of the newly arrived persons who have no prior engagement with it, thus testifying to the power of institutions to provoke certain kinds of behavior. The psychiatric OPD of a general hospital, in contrast, elicits a quite different set of practical responses. Yet, in both cases we seem to be dealing with the co-constitutive nature of experiences, ideas, and institutions that establish a more or less consistent system of ideas and practices with respect to the world and human beings' place in it.

On this basis Quack goes on to argue that the relevant cultural knowledge and practices, partly understood (following Charles Taylor) as an unformulated "background," are very important in understanding behaviors and beliefs regarding "possession." This background is discussed by Taylor in terms of "porous selves," a concept that is compared to Marriott's concept of "dividuals." Yet, while both models can be seen to account for specific forms of subjectivity conducive of "possession" experiences, Quack argues that

Marriott's and Taylor's insights have to be unhinged from their larger theoretical frameworks, and that they should be complemented with recent anthropological insights on the topic of "learning possession." The triad of ideas, practices, and institutions is not as static, mono-lithic, or culture-bound as Marriott and Taylor suggest, and accord-ingly Quack outlines why it is in many ways problematic to speak of Indian "dividuality" or "porous selves" living in an "enchanted world." Drawing on his ethnographic study of members of the ratio-nalist organization ANiS (*Andhashraddha Nirmulan Samiti* (Soci-ety for the Eradication of Superstition)), Quack argues that Indian rationalists do not fit into the wider cosmologies and social systems in which practices of possession are embedded. Moreover, given the reality of religious and medical pluralism and the diversity of lifestyles and influences in contemporary India and elsewhere, it is important not to generalize dualistic models and oppositions such as those of Marriott and Taylor too broadly. Studies of "health-seeking behavior" should therefore not begin with static binaries, but focus instead on how people (are forced to) make culturally informed choices on the basis of their embodied dispositions and on how they cultivate or struggle with different subjectivities. The coexistence and interplay between apparently contrasting kinds of subjectivities and dispositions cannot be captured by approaches that dichotomize between individuality and dividuality, enchantment and disenchant-ment. The challenge is to theorize the ways in which many people approach *Balaji* and also visit psychiatrists.

In the chapter that follows, Francis Zimmermann combines anthropology and Indology, focusing on the language used in medi-cal discourse in the context of practice, and thus offers a fresh per-spective on the dualisms of "East/West" and "medicine/alternative medicine." He argues that the reasons underlying choices for "alter-native" treatment are misunderstood by social scientists as attempts to resist conventional (bio)medicine. Neither can the division of labor between alternative and conventional medicine, or the opposi-tion between the medical practices and scientific beliefs of doctors, on the one hand, and "alternative" private beliefs and practices of patients and doctors, on the other, be explained simply in terms of an ideological division between "traditional" and "modern."

This argument is substantiated by a discussion of what it means when an Indian doctor comforts a patient by saying that the outcome of the treatment depends on "God's will." The doctor seems to be superimposing a "clinical theodicy" (Bharadwaj 2008) on clinical rationality, but Zimmermann argues that "God" in such contexts calls for a specific gloss, which is found in the classical Ayurvedic concept of *daiva* (destiny). According to Zimmermann, this term belongs to the physical dimension of the world and actually translates a classical doctrine of therapeutic prognosis, the structure of which is very different from the Western scheme. As he puts it, in the face of this classical doctrine, Broom's dichotomy between the rational, which would characterize conventional medicine, and the metaphysical, which would characterize traditional and alternative ideologies of health and disease, does not hold. There is no fixed dichotomy but rather a context-sensitive combination of three dimensions.

In his attempt to outline the dimensions central to classical Ayurveda and Indian philosophy and cosmology, Zimmermann is inspired by Marriott's (1976, 1990) ethnosociological approach to traditional Hindu taxonomies. Zimmermann differentiates between (a) the dimension of physics and time, or *daiva;* (b) the dimension of ethics and human agency, or *sattva;* and (c) the logical dimension of "logic" and "junctions," *yukti* and yoga. Zimmermann relates these three categories, respectively, to Marriott's three constitutive dimensions of the Hindu world: "mixing versus unmixing," "unmarking versus marking," and "unmatching versus matching," all of which are "devoid of any spiritual or spiritualistic connotations."

Zimmermann argues that these insights concerning the nonmetaphysical interrelatedness of different dimensions of physics, morality, logics, and social relations, alongside other crucial elements of classical Ayurveda, are "lost in translation" when reformulated in English. Focusing on doctor-patient encounters, he emphasizes the plurality of addressees attending the Ayurvedic consultation where the patient's individuality could be "dissolved as it were into the anonymity of humors and complaints" and argues that "the fragmentation of medical conversation into fixed phrases and lists of items emphasize(s) the dependency of the individual patient on her family circle." He emphasizes the way in which language is essential to world making through Hindu categories by elaborating the central position of verbal interaction in South Asian institutions and practices. When an Ayurvedic doctor uses Sanskrit words to formulate a diagnosis, a prognosis, and a prescription for the benefit of an individual patient, "categories are words meant to be enunciated by speakers expressing thought for action." He also argues that the doctor's attitude toward the patient, based as it is on the recognition that he is "both the same with, and different from, the self beyond death or the skin," implies a form of medical ethics that is central to the humoral system of Ayurveda. According to Zimmermann, this is similar to what Marriott calls "dividuality," the existence of a bond of nature, the commonality between all creatures, the recognition of which enables the ethical principle of friendliness (*maitrī*) in the strict sense of the term.

Zimmermann concludes by looking at how classical Ayurveda addresses "cancer." Once again employing Marriott's categories, he argues that cancer, within this rearticulated schema, should be seen as resulting from a combination of marking (pollution and tumescence), mixing (pervasion), and unmatching (division and disorder), thereby showing how "boundaries are blurred between health and disease, between medicines and poisons, and between life and death," given that in this perspective the world is "essentially dividual (or mixed), unbalanced (or marked) and chaotic (or unmatched)."

Another prism that captures the hegemony of the biomedical model is pregnancy and childbirth. The successful medicalization of childbirth in the West, and the continuing attempts to do so by modernizing states the world over so as to reduce infant and maternal mortality, is a prime example of the metamorphosis of a domestic and communal event into a medical one. In the chapter following Zimmermann's, Harish Naraindas argues that along with childhood vaccinations, pregnancy is one of the most "successful" examples of medicalization, given that around 97 percent of women in the United States and Germany continue to give birth in medical institutions, despite sustained attempts by small but vocal groups of home-birth advocates to convince them to do otherwise. This drive to institutionalize or hospitalize birth has some similarities to the nascent drive in India to institutionalize the "mentally ill" (see Basu this volume and Quack 2012). The attempt to reduce or eliminate home births in those places where they continue, based on the assumption that institutional deliveries reduce infant and maternal mortality, is simultaneously an attempt to replicate a Western norm worldwide. The irony is that this institutionalization or hospitalization of birth is often resisted by educated Western women, who see this and related medical procedures as disempowering, unsafe, and altogether unnecessary; or as "rituals" rather than responses to need, with dubious histories and problematic consequences (Davis-Floyd 1990; Selvaraj et al. 2006; Naraindas 2008).

Based primarily on a single retrospective narrative of an educated, urban, middle-class Indian woman's attempt to circumvent a hospitalized birth, Harish Naraindas shows how such an attempt is fraught with risks of stigma, deformity, and death. The expectant mother is forced to shuttle between her *vaidya* (Ayurvedic physician) and her gynecologist, since her *vaidya*, who is the preferred physician and the person with whom the mother would rather deliver her child, is not in a position to offer this facility. This results in her running a dual course between two physicians and two systems, with one of them (namely Ayurveda) being frowned upon by family and friends, either as a form of quackery, or as too risky for an event as grave and important as pregnancy, thus forcing her to hide from her gynecologist the fact that she consults an Ayurvedic physician. The result is a minefield that the prospective mother is called upon to negotiate, since she is privy neither to a single source of expert authority, nor to a *vade mecum* to help her negotiate sticky situations.

Naraindas uses this narrative to question several paradigms that have been proposed for understanding doctor-patient interactions or health-seeking behavior, *none of which* have been forged in the crucible of competing theories of disease or modes of expertise, but rather as consequences of the presumed opposition between the expertise of the doctor and the culture of the patient, or between disease (the provenance of the doctor) and illness (the experience of the patient). He argues that this opposition, which has bedeviled medical anthropology, presupposes that there is but one universal nosology and one universal definition of disease, based, tacitly, on a universal doctor and a universal (biomedical) episteme with its attendant ontology. What we witness instead in this narrative is a patient/person who attempts to exercise agency between *at least* two competing epistemes, neither of which is able in every situation to resolve her existential crisis.

Naraindas's chapter is thus a prime example of a contested conversation between systems and (as we have pointed out above) calls into question not only the notion of pluralism but also ready and easy notions of South Asian syncretism (Leslie 1976), along with notions of hybridity and their cognate concepts of domestication and vernacularization, to show that one needs to go beyond these ready and easy notions, and think rather of "conversations" between systems marked by severe asymmetries, which often lead to charges of quackery and criminalization, as Adams (2002) has shown for the case of Tibetan medicine in its encounter with biomedicine or, as Naraindas argues elsewhere, to forms of creolization (Naraindas 2014).

This theme of *conversations* between systems is pursued in the next chapter by Helene Basu by returning to the theme of possession. Unlike Quack's chapter, where temple and clinic are kept apart, with each "asking" of its clientele a certain disposition that is particular to its site, in Basu's chapter we see the clinic intruding into the shrine under the aegis of the state. This intrusion of the psychiatric clinic into the *Mira Data Dargāh* Sufi shrine in Gujarat, brought about by the public health department under its "*Davā* and *Duā*" (medicine and prayer) program, may be seen as a variant of the attempt to "mainstream" (a euphemism for absorbing, negating, appropriating, or expropriating) such healing shrines (Quack 2012). This mainstreaming was prompted by the famous Erwadi tragedy of 2001, where persons chained to trees and other structures near a Sufi shrine in Tamilnadu perished in a fire. This led parts of the media to launch a tirade against such "barbaric practices," and the Supreme Court, through a *suo motu* motion, passed a judgment requiring the Government of India to take cognizance of the situation and act on it. While some members of the public health department would have liked to "act" by shutting down shrines like the one researched by Basu, this might have led to a "communal problem" or could have been perceived as an anti-Muslim act in a state that is currently seen in the national media as being discriminatory and hostile toward Muslims. Hence, the *Davā* and *Duā* program appears to be a compromise dreamed up by the state and a local NGO to help the "patients" (actually they are pilgrims or supplicants) gain access to a "proper" diagnosis and "real" (psychopharmaceutical) medicines, in addition to prayer and healing rituals. This has led to a kind of "enforced pluralization" of healing practices at the shrine.

Basu describes both kinds of treatment through a detailed ethnography. On the one side are the *khādim* or "priests" and the pilgrims

17

approaching them for help, both of whose practices and perspectives are illustrated through several case studies. These contrast with "the culture of the psychiatric project," and the role of the *khādim* in accommodating it. It is apparent that they themselves are divided on this issue, with some of them supporting it, while others resist it (which may simply mean not sending their patients to the psychiatrists). Some *khādim* opposed the project on the grounds that its very existence called the sacrality and power of the *dargāh* into question, while others supported it, not only because they saw the presence of the psychiatrists and the state as an opportunity, since it lent further credence to the shrine as a place of healing, but also because they did indeed believe that there were certain mental diseases more appropriately treated by psychiatrists than with religious therapy.

Basu argues that there are different ways in which the notions *davā* and *duā* can be understood. *Duā* roughly means "prayer" in a Muslim context, but can also connote religious treatment as opposed to *davā* (medicine), i.e., the practices of biomedicine. For those who launched the *davā* and *duā* project, *davā* refers to psychotropic medications necessary for mentally ill people, whereas *duā* refers to religious practices that may be helpful as techniques ancillary to such medications. What is special about this particular context is that the psychiatric discourse is subordinated to the religious one, both spatio-architecturally (it is located within the precincts of the shrine) and practically (most pilgrims visit the psychiatrists as an afterthought, or merely out of curiosity). Basu shows this through case studies in which the patients consult the resident psychiatrist at the behest of the *pīr* (the saint of the shrine, who may appear either to the sufferer or his attendant in a dream), or through the intermediary of the *khādim*, who speaks on his behalf. She argues that internal pluralization, being enforced on the shrine by the state, places new demands on practitioners, psychiatrists, as well as the *khādim*, to mutually acknowledge each other's understandings of mental disorder and methods of healing. There is however some doubt about how far these "acknowledgments" go, and to what degree we have here an example of two very different systems (one medical, one more comprehensive) operating side by side at one and the same place. "Medical pluralism" did prevail within the precincts of the shrine but, as Basu points out, "pluralizing the institutional space of a mental hospital by granting a place to ritual specialists performing rituals for hospitalized patients" would not have been possible. Such is the nature of asymmetry.

While Basu's chapter wrestles with an enforced pluralism at state behest, the next chapter, by Willliam S. Sax and Hari Bhaskar, argues that Ayurvedic medicines and religious techniques need not be mutually exclusive. Here we see the coming together of what may be called the "physical" and the "metaphysical" under a single overarching system, which may cause conceptual problems for the outside observer but seems quite unproblematic for the healers. Sax and Bhaskar's ethnography of a well-known family of high-caste Nambudiri Brahmins in Malappuram district, Kerala, overturns the usual depiction of such healers as being of lower caste, and also bears witness to an admixture of realms when they describe how healers "employ a unique mix of religious techniques with mainstream Ayurvedic ones."

They exorcize demons, but also prescribe modern Ayurvedic medicines; their practice resembles in some ways a Hindu temple, but in other ways an Ayurvedic clinic; they use internet advertising and participate in a complex, modern system of referrals among medical doctors and Ayurvedic physicians; but people close to them attribute their success to their ascetic lifestyle.

The authors ask whether this mix of "scientific" and "nonscientific" therapies makes the healers "premodern, nonmodern, modernizing, hybrid, or something else," and they argue that posing this question helps us to better understand how the ideology of modernity distorts our understanding of nonbiomedical healing systems. They claim that modernization theory is based upon many of the dualisms that we listed above. In fact, one can safely say that without those dualisms as both prop and goal, where recalcitrant populations worldwide are expected to move from the deficient "premodern" term to the superior "modern" one, modernization theory would collapse. Hence, they briefly summarize modernization theory and its critics, underscore its importance, describe and analyze the healers' practice in light of these aspects, and conclude that the healers' mixture of "modern" and "nonmodern" medicine is not as unusual as it perhaps seems.

Such mixtures are characteristic, they argue, not only of Asian medical practice, but also of "modern" medicine in Europe (cf. Naraindas 2011a, 2011b) and North America. This claim is borne out by the fact that the same Ayurveda, when it travels abroad and attempts to establish itself as a professional practice within a regulatory scheme where biomedicine is dominant, manages to straddle two different worlds: the biomedicalized world of modern Ayurveda with its regulatory regimes, and the spiritualized world of European Ayurveda with its informal networks.

Mixing the two together, says Maya Warrier in her examination of Ayurveda in Britain, leads not to closure and streamlining but heterogeneity and experimentation. Her argument is based on an examination of the history and role of the Ayurvedic Practitioners Association (APA), currently the single most important Ayurvedic professional body in the U.K. The main focus of the chapter is the effects of professionalization due to the government's regulatory initiatives on Ayurveda in Britain in general and the APA in particular. Warrier argues that professionalization did not lead to a "domestication" of this medical tradition in its British manifestation. On the contrary, the APA, though it has a standardized core, was able to uphold the "informal, spontaneous, creative and non-medicalized networks and lifeworlds upon which it draws for its vitality." She presents a detailed study of how the APA was able to hold its informal networks and formal institutional aspects in creative tension with one another and how it continues to embrace considerable plurality and diversity in worldviews, practices, and modes of therapy and treatment.

In a historical overview Warrier outlines how, after the impressive growth of Ayurveda in the U.K., the British government was forced to take this medical tradition seriously, despite considerable suspicion. This became necessary particularly after Ayurveda was recognized by the U.K. government (following intensive lobbying on the part of practitioners) as a tradition for which there was some scientific evidence of its health benefits (real or potential). This recognition meant that Ayurveda had to submit to the requirements of a proposed framework of statutory regulation for particular complementary and alternative medical systems. The APA was founded to secure Ayurveda's interests within the new regulatory framework. With respect to the contemporary practice of Ayurveda in the U.K., Warrier identifies two distinct strands. On the one hand is the "medicalized" (biomedicalized) version of this tradition that resembles

Ayurveda as it is mainly taught and studied in Indian colleges and universities. On the other hand are the homegrown, "spiritualized" versions of Ayurveda, where practitioners combine what they learn with lifeworlds characterized by spiritual seeking and esoteric meaning. "Spirituality as understood here is closely linked with notions of self-responsibility, and self-transformation and self-empowerment through self-knowledge."

Given these two versions, there were initially problems finding representatives who were respected by both sides, and formulating standardized processes and procedures for contemporary Ayurveda in the U.K. Still, Warrier argues that the APA managed to combine these two versions under one institutional roof as well as to engage with the government, its regulatory initiatives, and other groups in the CAM sector. By drawing upon "spirituality" the APA was able to develop robust informal, creative, and heterogenous networks in the CAM sector and the esoteric milieu interested in holistic health. According to Warrier, the APA fits into this milieu as a moral community endorsing the values commonly attributed to "spirituality" such as self-understanding, self-awareness, and self-responsibility. Further characteristics include the APA's position as a "nodal institution operating within a vast informal network connecting up a range of sociocultural traditions, holistic health therapies, guru-led organizations, networks centering on different forms of popular psychology, meditation groups, and green activism." Warrier concludes that the APA has thus far succeeded in straddling a healthy middle ground between the regulatory constraints of the mainstream and the creative freedom of the fringe. By holding its formal institutional aspects and its informal networks in creative tension with each other the APA has not been domesticated, but has instead enhanced its own processes of creativity, heterogeneity, and experimentation.

Coda: Contestations and the Blurring of Boundaries

All the chapters in this volume wrestle with how health seeking takes place within a globalized and blurred milieu, how and why certain kinds of health practices or dispositions have been produced and naturalized, and what happens when sufferers, providers, and practitioners attempt to avoid, resist, transform, or even transcend them. They draw explicitly or implicitly on the interrelations of beliefs, practices, and formal institutions. While some observe self-reinforcing loops among institutions, practices, and concepts, others focus on the ways in which people sometimes seek to bypass, circumvent, or even transcend the dominant ideologies of their cultures as represented in the main institutions of health care. Finally, the looping, along with the various attempts at circumvention, takes place in systems that are marked by numerous asymmetries: not only between different systems, but also between healers and sufferers, medical and metaphysical forms of curing, public and private providers, "East" and "West," "mind" and "body." All the chapters bear witness to what sometimes appears to be a Manichean struggle between asymmetrical oppositions that structure the pedagogy and practice of contemporary modes of healing. Depending on the context, the different approaches explore the emergence of boundaries (Kirmayer), their blurring (Sax and Bhaskar), or their redrawing, especially when patients attempt to circumvent the seemingly dominant system in their health-seeking behavior (Naraindas). This seems to lead at times to a reversal of the asymmetry and the privileging of the second of the two terms (Basu, Naraindas, Sax and Bhaskar), though the end result is often a kind of negotiated settlement, or the interweaving of a formal requirement and an informal one (Warrier). Finally, some contributions show the inadequacy of well-established boundaries with respect to certain groups (Quack) or healing practices (Zimmermann). But in all these cases, neither the relations between the various systems of healing, nor patients' choices with respect to them, nor the processes of historical and cultural change, can be understood without taking into account ideas, institutions, and practices regarding health, disease, and well-being, where the dualism of mind and body, with its several homologues, continues to structure the discourse and practice of medicine.

Notes

1. Good examples are the notion of the "pugilistic habitus," as elaborated in a study of a boxing gym in a black ghetto of Chicago, by Loïc Wacquant (2004), and Joseph Alter's *The Wrestler's Body* (1992), which is a study of a wrestling *akhara* in India.

References

Adams, Vincanne. 2002. "Randomised Controlled Crime: Postcolonial Sciences in Alternative Medicine Research." *Social Studies of Science* 32(5-6): 659–690.

Alter, Joseph. 1992. *The Wrestler's Body: Identity and Ideology in North India.* Berkeley: University of California Press.

Attewell, Guy. 2007. *Refiguring Unani Tibb: Plural Healing in Late Colonial India.* New Delhi: Orient Longman.

Banerjee, Madhulika. 2009. *Power, Knowledge, Medicine: Ayurvedic Pharmaceuticals at Home and in the World.* Hyderabad: Orient BlackSwan.

Bharadwaj, Aditya. 2008. "Biosocialities and Biocrossings: Encounters with Assisted Conception and Embryonic Stem Cells in India." In *Biosocialities, Genetics and the Social Sciences: Making Biologies and Identities,* ed. Sahra Gibbon and Carlos Novas. London: Routledge, 98–116.

Bode, Maarten. 2008. *Taking Traditional Knowledge to the Market: The Modern Image of the Ayurvedic and Unani Industry, 1980—2000.* Hyderabad: Orient Longman.

Bourdieu, Pierre. 1998. *Practical Reason: On the Theory of Action.* Stanford: Stanford University Press.

Canguilhem, Georges. 1978. *On the Normal and the Pathological.* Boston: The D. Riedel Publishing Company.

Davis-Floyd, Robbie E. 1990. "The Role of Obstetrical Rituals in the Resolution of Cultural Anomaly." *Social Science & Medicine* 31(2): 175–189.

Ecks, Stefan. 2005. "Pharmaceutical Citizenship: Antidepressant Marketing and the Promise of Demarginalization in India." *Anthropology & Medicine* 12(3): 239–254.

Ecks, Stefan, and Soumita Basu. 2009. "The Unlicensed Lives of Antidepressants in India: Generic Drugs, Unqualified Practitioners and Floating Prescriptions." *Transcultural Psychiatry* 46(1): 86–106.

Elias, Norbert. 1939. *Über den Prozeß der Zivilisation: Soziogenetische und psychogenetische Untersuchungen.* Basel: Haus zum Falken.

Ernst, Waltraud. 1991. "Racial, Social and Cultural Factors in the Development of a Colonial Institution: The Bombay Lunatic Asylum 1670-1858." *Internationales Asienforum* 22(34): 61–80.

Farmer, Paul. 2003. "On Suffering and Structural Violence: Social and Economic Rights in the Global Era." In *Pathologies of Power: Health, Human Rights, and the New War on the Poor,* ed. Paul Farmer. Berkeley: University of California Press, 29–50.

Foucault, Michel. 1973. *The Birth of the Clinic: An Archaeology of Medical Perception.* London: Tavistock.

Hacking, Ian. 1995. *Rewriting the Soul: Multiple Personality and the Sciences of Memory.* Princeton: Princeton University Press.

———. 1999. *The Social Construction of What?* Cambridge, M.A.: Harvard University Press.

Halliburton, Murphy. 2009. *Mudpacks and Prozac: Experiencing Ayurvedic, Biomedical and Religious Healing*. Walnut Creek: Left Coast Press.

Kirmayer, Laurence, and Norman Sartorius. 2007. "Cultural Models and Somatic Syndromes." *Psychosomatic Medicine* 69(9): 832–840.

Lang, Claudia, and Eva Jansen. 2013. "Appropriating Depression: Biomedicalizing Ayurvedic Psychiatry in Kerala, India." *Medical Anthropology* 32(1): 25–45.

Langford, Jean, M. 2002. *Fluent Bodies: Ayurvedic Remedies for Postcolonial Imbalance*. Durham: Duke University Press.

Latour, Bruno. 1993. *We Have Never Been Modern*. Cambridge, M.A.: Harvard University Press.

Leslie, Charles. 1976. *Asian Medical Systems: A Comparative Study*. Berkeley: University of California Press.

Leslie, C., and A. Young. 1992. *Paths to Asian Medical Knowledge*. Berkeley: University of California Press.

Marriott, McKim. 1976. "Hindu Transactions: Diversity without Dualism." In *Transaction and Meaning: Directions in the Anthropology of Exchange and Symbolic Behaviour*, ed. Bruce Kapferer. Philadelphia: Institute for the Study of Human Issues, 109–142.

———. 1990. "Constructing an Indian Ethnosociology." In *India Through Hindu Categories*, ed. McKim Marriott. New Delhi: Sage Publications, 1–39.

Mauss, Marcel. 1935. "Les Techniques du Corps." *Journal de Psychologie* 32(3-4): 271–293. Reprinted in Marcel Mauss. 1968. *Sociologie et Anthropologie*. Paris: Presses Universitaires de France, 364–386.

Naraindas, Harish. 2006. "Of Spineless Babies and Folic Acid: Evidence and Efficacy in Biomedicine and Ayurvedic Medicine." *Social Science & Medicine* 62(11): 2658–2669.

———. 2008. "Mainstreaming AYUSH and Ayushing Obstetrics." *Health for the Millions* 34(2-3): 33–37.

———. 2011a. "Of Relics, Body Parts and Laser Beams: The German Heilpraktiker and his Ayurvedic Spa." *Anthropology and Medicine* 18(1): 67–86.

———. 2011b. "Korallen, Chipkarten, Medizinischen Informationen und die Jungfrau Maria: Heilpraktiker in Deutschland und die Aneignung der Ayurveda Therapie." *Zeitschrift für Ethnologie* 136: 93–114.

———. 2014. "Nosopolitics: Epistemic Mangling and the Creolization of Contemporary Ayurveda." In *Medical Pluralism and Homeopathy in India and Germany (1810-2010): A Comparison of Practices*, ed. Martin Dinges. *Medizin, Gesellschaft und Geschichte, (MedGG-Beiheft 50), Jahrbuch des Instituts für Geschichte der Medizin der Robert Bosch Stiftung*. Stuttgart: Franz Steiner Verlag, 105–136.

Quack, Johannes. 2012. "Ignorance and Utilization: Mental Health Care Outside the Purview of the Indian State." *Anthropology & Medicine* 19(3): 277–290.

———. 2013. "'What Do I Know?' Scholastic Fallacies and Pragmatic Religiosity in Mental Health-Seeking Behaviour in India." *Mental Health, Religion & Culture* 16(4): 403–418.

Reddy, Sita. 2002. "Asian Medicine in America: The Ayurvedic Case." *Annals of the American Academy of Political and Social Science: Global Perspectives on Complementary and Alternative Medicine* 583 (September): 97–121.

———. 2004. "The Politics and Poetics of 'Magazine Medicine': New Age Ayurveda in the Print Media." In *The Politics of Healing: Histories of Alternative Medicine in Twentieth-Century North America,* ed. Robert Johnston. London: Routledge, 207–231.

Robertson, Roland. 1995. "Glocalization: Time-Space and Homogeneity-Heterogeneity." In *Global Modernities,* ed. Mike Featherstone, Scott Lash, and Roland Robertson. London: Sage Publications, 25–44.

Sébastia, Brigitte. 2009. *Restoring Mental Health in India: Pluralistic Therapies and Concepts.* New Delhi: Oxford University Press.

Selvaraj, Alphonse, A. Chitra, and S. Parvathy. 2006 *Episiotomy: Real Need or Ritual?* Poonamalee, Chennai: Institute of Public Health.

Sivaramakrishnan, Kavita. 2006. *Old Potions, New Bottle: Recasting Indigenous Medicine in Colonial Punjab (1850–1945).* New Delhi: Orient Longman.

Wacquant, Loïc. 2004. *Body and Soul: Ethnographic Notebooks of an Apprentice-Boxer.* New York: Oxford University Press.

Wujastyk, Dagmar, and Frederick M. Smith. 2008. *Modern and Global Ayurveda: Pluralism and Paradigms.* Albany: State University of New York.

Young, Allan. 1995. *Harmony of Illusions: Inventing Posttraumatic Stress Disorder.* Princeton: Princeton University Press.

Zimmermann, Francis (1992). "Gentle Purge: The Flower Power of Ayurveda." In *Paths to Asian Medical Knowledge,* ed. Charles Leslie and Allan Young. Berkeley: University of California Press, 209–223.

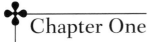

Chapter One
Medicines of the Imagination
Cultural Phenomenology,
Medical Pluralism, and the
Persistence of Mind-Body Dualism

Laurence J. Kirmayer

Introduction

The colonialism that spread Western medicine throughout the
world generally saw other medical systems as primitive and crudely
empirical, or else as thoroughly irrational, based on magic and
superstition. Western medicine claimed to be grounded in science
and represented one of the chief fruits of Enlightenment rationality. Traditional systems of healing were marginalized or studied as
curiosities that might be mined for ethnobotanical knowledge or
to reveal the social and psychological functions of ritual and symbolic action. This epistemological divide was gendered, racialized,
and hierarchical, with northern European male styles of explanation, justification, and comportment the explicit standard against
which other practices and traditions were measured and usually
found wanting. This colonial machinery and dominant system of
values, however, did not prevent the constant exchange, circulation, mutual transformation, and proliferation of diverse kinds of
medicine (Ernst 2007), so that we increasingly live in a global agora
with highly pluralistic systems of medicine in every urban center. It
is in the context of this ongoing circulation and competition among
different systems of medicine and their associated epistemologies
and ontologies that biomedical institutions have framed other

approaches—whether rooted in venerable historical traditions or recent, hybrid inventions—as Complementary and Alternative Medicine (CAM). The hope expressed in this labeling of CAM is that an ecological niche can be carved out that respects the fact of medical pluralism while allowing some measure of regulation that will protect the dominance of biomedicine as the recognized mainstream rather than just another alternative.

Indeed, CAM is part of larger global economic, knowledge, and discursive systems and has grown hand in hand with the expansion of biomedicine (Lyng 2010). This reflects the use of similar business, professional, and institutional strategies but also a deliberate engagement with critiques of the limits biomedicine as currently practiced. Contemporary holistic, alternative, and complementary medicines promise to repair a split between mind and body that has a long history in Western traditions. Much popular writing on health, along with the work of many social scientists, has described non-Western medical systems as inherently integrative, avoiding the conceptual dichotomy between imaginary maladies and real diseases that plagues biomedicine, vexing doctors and patients alike. But this portrait of non-Western ("Eastern," Asian, African, indigenous) medicines as integrative or holistic is usually based on sympathetic readings of esoteric texts that emphasize metaphors of balance, harmony, and cosmological order. In actual practice, many healing traditions make distinctions between illnesses of the body and afflictions that seem to primarily affect the person's cognitive and social functioning. This distinction may reflect pan-cultural universals in the phenomenology of illness experience. At the same time, cultural differences in the underlying ontologies of illness causation and experience lead to important differences in how afflictions are understood and treated. Even when an illness has somatic manifestations, its causes may be sought in a sociomoral or spiritual realm. This chapter considers the origins, persistence, and pervasiveness of dualistic thinking in medicine and offers some reflections on the rationalities of biomedicine as well as complementary and alternative medicines. Understanding the cultural phenomenological roots and epistemic consequences of the ontologies of diverse healing systems can shed light on the politics and pragmatics of medical pluralism in contemporary societies (Kirmayer 2012).

Dualism and the History of the Imagination in Western Medicine

Although Western mind-body dualism is conventionally blamed on René Descartes, its roots can be traced in far earlier distinctions between body and psyche in Greek philosophy (Claus 1981; Solmsen 1983).[1] And while many other medical traditions do not make the same ontological distinctions between diseases of the body and afflictions of the soul or spirit, there is a sense in which mind/body dualism is based on a deeper and perhaps universal phenomenological distinction between the body as corruptible and mortal and the mind as the seat of a consciousness capable of imagining its own immortality (Kirmayer 1988; Lambek 1998). While the range and mobility of imagination are often constrained by pain, nausea, and other preemptive bodily sensations that arrest attention and constrict awareness, imagination can break free of these constraints to roam widely and ascend to the higher realms represented in cultural and spiritual ontologies (Shulman 2012).

In the medicine of the early Renaissance, imagination occupied a central role (Fischer-Homberger 1979). For Paracelsus (Theophrastus Bombastus von Hohenheim, 1493/94–1541), imagination was a "celestial" (supernatural) force that acts directly on the material world to refashion matter in its image. This could occur within the womb when a woman's imagination left its impress on her unborn child, but also throughout the course of life whenever strong emotion or volition converted itself into something physical or into a spirit that can act on matter. "All action is visualised by Paracelsus as flowing from an act of imagination—a process not connected with formal logical reasoning, but with the spirit-conscious or subconscious" (Pagel 1982: 111). This view of imagination was rooted in a dualistic ontology in which human beings have two bodies, one visible and the other invisible—and the invisible body is the more powerful one:

> There are two realms into which diseases can penetrate and spread. The first is that of matter, that is to say, the body; it is here that all diseases lurk and dwell . . . the other realm is not material, it is the spirit of the body, which lives in it intangible and invisible, and which can suffer from exactly the same diseases as the body. But because the body has no share in this life, it is the *ens spirituale*, the spiritual active principle, from

which the disease springs. . . . Therefore there are two kinds of disease:
the spiritual and the material. (Paracelsus, in: Jacobi, 1988: 75)

Similar distinctions between the visible and the invisible or intan-
gible aspects of the body, along with the notion that what is more
subtle is also more powerful, can be found in classical Hindu philosophical texts (see, for example, Daniel 1984: 233ff.; Doniger 1997).
Beyond this apparent duality, however, Paracelsus asserted the fundamental unity of spirit and body, of macrocosm and microcosm. He
did so through a reification of the spirit and an arrogation of divine
powers for the human faculties of imagination. He supported this
with a style of argument that moved directly from analogy to identity, literalizing metaphors to elide distinctions and fuse disparate
realms (Vickers 1984). The reification of metaphor characteristic of
alchemical thinking allowed imagination full sway. But, in an effort
to turn poetic analogy into technical knowledge, Paracelsus coined
neologisms to cover his intuitive leaps so that he could make the
self-mystifying claim, "it is a lack of skill to use *metaphora* in medicine and nothing but an error to give names metaphorically" (Paracelsus, quoted in Temkin 1952: 216). This denial of the metaphoric
logic of his reasoning was part of Paracelsus's rhetorical claim to
truth as the foundation of his medical practice.

Paracelsus claims and, indeed, his whole style of argument were
attacked by the early figures of the scientific Enlightenment (Vickers
1984). For Frances Bacon and other critics, Paracelsus constructed
spurious arguments by ignoring levels of language and meaningful
distinctions. To put it in contemporary terms, reason consisted in
maintaining an awareness of one's models as metaphors and being
ready to cast them aside when an analogy broke down because it
diverged from empirical evidence. This gradually emerging rationalism and scientific empiricism forced one to recognize and respect
the limits of the metaphorical imagination.

Enlightenment thinkers feared the corrupting effects of imagination because they saw a real danger in losing oneself in illusory
images and thoughts (Daston 1998). Imagination had a fearsome
power to conjure misleading worlds that could drive a person mad.
Clarity and correctness of facts depended on reining in this profli-
gacy. Of course, imagination was essential to apprehend nature, but
it had to be subdued and constrained by reason (whence Francisco

Goya: *The Sleep of Reason Produces Monsters*). For Voltaire, healthy imagination was "active"—engaged with and driven by reason—while passive imagination could lead to pathology and moral failure. This emerging epistemology reflected phenomenological distinctions but only gradually developed a firmer footing through a set of scientific methodologies.

The investigation and ultimate debunking the claims of the physician and popular healer Franz Anton Mesmer by the French Royal Commissions, toward the end of the eighteenth century, was an important turning point in the medical history of the imagination (Darnton 1968; Gauld 1992). Mesmer understood his healing method as the control of the physical forces of animal magnetism. Driven more by political than epistemological worries, the Royal Commissions aimed to examine the reality of Mesmer's notions of magnetic fluids and forces of "animal magnetism." The commissioners were less concerned with healing efficacy than with Mesmer's claims to have identified a fundamental force, reasoning that if the force did not exist, any claim for specific healing efficacy could be dismissed. Their method of inquiry was empirical and experimental: they subjected themselves to mesmeric treatments and conducted blinded tests of the effects of animal magnetism—trying to avoid being influenced by suggestions. The conclusion: "Mesmer's fluid did not exist; the convulsions and other effects of mesmerizing could be attributed to the overheated imaginations of the mesmerists" (Darnton 1968: 64). Imagination was recognized as being powerful enough to cause the dramatic swoons and fits of Mesmer's treatments and subsequent claims of cure, but this power was due to the suggestibility of certain individuals (McConkey and Perry 2002).

While the account of the Royal Commission could have been read as testimony to the importance of imagination, the fact that sober scientists did not experience the same dramatic effects directed attention to the gullibility of people with "over-heated imaginations." Although couched in the language of science, mesmerism was revealed to be pseudoscience. Despite this debunking, mesmerism enjoyed renewed popularity in Victorian England, France, and the United States, but the association with irrationality set the stage for its decline (Fuller 1982; Winter 1998; Schmit 2005). In colonial India, the successful applications of mesmerism for surgical anesthesia by the British surgeon John Esdaile were the subject of much interest but were taken by many as evidence for Indian irrationality and "native superstition" (Ernst 2004: 64). The ultimate demise of mesmerism came with the appropriation of the unconscious by psychoanalysis with its assertion of the capacity of the rational ego, guided by the objectifying gaze of the analyst, to make sense of the individual's inconsistencies, resistances, dissociative gaps, and self-deceptions (Ellenberger 1970; Zaretsky 2004).

Subsequent attention to the phenomena of hypnosis and hysteria did not focus on understanding the faculty of imagination but on the nature of suggestible individuals, who were viewed as gullible and histrionic, beset by traumatic memories and intrapsychic conflict, or, in the work of Jean Martin Charcot and others, as suffering from pathologies of the nervous system (Micale 1995). This association of imagination with certain personality traits or types continues to the present in studies of hypnotizability, suggestibility, and the "fantasy-prone" personality (Hilgard 1979; Lynn and Rhue 1986). What was lost in this shift toward individual traits and vulnerabilities was the recognition of the power and ubiquity of imagination in everyday life and the likelihood that everyone, under suitable circumstances consonant with their core beliefs and commitments, is suggestible. This equation of imagination with gullibility or unusual susceptibility to social influence meant that a basic human faculty was displaced from its central position in our picture of the mind and increasingly viewed as both trivial and embarrassing, if not dangerous. In so doing, the gap was widened between the mental processes that give meaning to illness experience and the physiological mechanisms that give rise to disease. This ontological distinction would be reinforced in nineteenth-century medicine by the epistemic distinction between subjective symptoms and objective signs of disease that could be confirmed by physical examination and, ultimately, by autopsy (Sullivan 1986; Foucault 1994).

Pragmatics of Belief in Healing Practices

Contemporary biomedicine is heir to the scientific rationalism that displaced and demoted the faculty of imagination. Biomedicine claims the rational, real, and material for its dominion, and consigns alternative medicine to the realm of the irrational and insubstantial. This does not mean, however, that such "alternative" practices are marginal in either cultural or economic terms. In 2005, people in the United States spent more than $27 billion on complementary and alternative medicine (CAM) (Carey 2006). Fully 62 percent of adults used at least one form of CAM in 2002 (Barnes et al. 2004). The most frequently used therapies were prayer, natural products, deep breathing exercises, meditation, chiropractic treatments, yoga, massage, and diet-based therapies. The most common problems brought to alternative practitioners are chronic conditions, especially pain and fatigue, for which there often is no clear medical explanation or effective treatment available. Far from being a set of marginal practices, this whole domain is big business for the companies that manufacture and market "natural" remedies and, in the aggregate, for the wide variety of local practitioners who offer treatment (Andrews et al. 2009; Vos and Brennan 2010). There are complex and often indirect links between global marketing efforts and local, independent practitioners who may be deeply ambivalent about the commercialization of treatments they dispense, even as they profit from and are dependent on these larger business activities.

This widespread use of alternative forms of healing reflects diverse systems of belief held with varying degrees of commitment and consistency—and different ways of life for which such practices may be central or peripheral, rigorously followed, or casually explored (Chaves 2010). In addition to the importance of prayer as part of Christian and other religious beliefs, there is a widespread attitude in North America that embraces non-Western forms of medicine as potentially superior to biomedical treatments, which, in turn, are viewed as unnatural, harsh, toxic, and accompanied by noxious side effects. Others—including many biomedical practitioners—express skepticism about alternative and complementary medicines based on the lack of evidence for their effectiveness (but see Nguyen et al. 2011).[2]

Although it is common to appeal to the antiquity of healing practices and to their persistence over long periods of time as evidence for their efficacy, the mere fact that a treatment is widely used does not demonstrate that it is efficacious or effective.[3] Indeed, many treatments are widely embraced despite clear evidence that they do not work any better than chance (or, at best, no better than any other nonspecific treatment or "placebo"). The conviction that ineffective remedies work may be based on common errors of reasoning or forms of "bounded rationality" (Kahneman 2003, 2011), which include the tendencies to interpret contiguity or correlation as causation, attribute cause to salient differences, and overgeneralize from small samples without comparison or control groups. All of these common biases and limitations in everyday reasoning join with wishful thinking to inflate the apparent efficacy of interventions. But these same styles of reasoning are also used in thinking about biomedical practices. So it is not merely an issue of thinking clearly but of allegiances and commitments to particular systems of knowledge or institutions that warrant specific healing practices. These allegiances may be explicit when they are part of the politics of individual and collective identity (e.g., a Jehovah's Witness who refuses blood transfusion, or a Christian Scientist who is committed to the healing power of spiritual transformation), or reflect strategic attempts at social positioning (as when someone asserts the value of a particular treatment because it allows them distance or independence from an institution or authority they mistrust), as well as more unconscious or implicit engagements that involve tacit participation in everyday practices that are part of a local community or lifeworld. Making commitments to, resisting, or rejecting a particular explanatory system may serve similar purposes of resource management, social positioning, and identity consolidation. The particular mix of these meanings and functions, however, is not entirely under the control of the individual, since the dominant cultural meanings of medical practices are shaped by larger social, economic, and political agendas.

Understanding the ways in which systems of medicine or healing practices come to seem attractive, authoritative, and potentially efficacious requires an appreciation for the different ways knowledge is produced, circulated, and employed by individuals in particular social and cultural contexts. In the contemporary world, most people have available a wide variety of healing knowledges and practices drawn from diverse traditions that have been detached from their larger conceptual frameworks, institutions, and communities of practice. What Levi-Straus called "bricolage" is the rule and this sort of handiwork serves both the personal search for effective remedies and local processes of forming alliances or communities of practice.

There are different levels of participation in a form of life ranging from temporarily making use of a frame of reference or metaphor that carries with it a set of implicit assumptions, to working with basic models or root metaphors that are used to structure all experience (and that exert ongoing influence because new information and experiences are interpreted through these frames), to making a commitment to an explicit identity or way of life that depends on specific assumptions. Modern subjects move between these levels of engagement, participating in them with varying degrees of intensity and conviction, based on their current needs, the demands of the institution itself, and the extent to which participation comes to play other roles in identity formation and social positioning. Thus, adopting a stance as a critical-minded skeptic or New Age enthusiast is not just a matter of aesthetics or intellectual proclivities but an opportunity to identify oneself as a certain kind of person, with a particular set of values that confer distinction and create belonging. As such, the move from one ideology or institution to another, or even from one style of reasoning and mode of illness explanation to another, is not just a matter of adopting a new discourse but of participating in a new identity and potential community.

No doubt, some of the appeal of traditional or alternative medicine comes from sheer exoticism or fascination with the foreign. Beyond this aesthetic attraction, arguments for the effectiveness of traditional or complementary medicine rest on styles of reasoning that variously invoke isolated cases or claims of individuals, the authority of tradition, the assumption that treatments that have survived a long time have proved their efficacy, and the fit of healing practices with other religious, spiritual, or philosophical convictions.

Of course, the most basic motivation for the use of any form of treatment is the hope for relief or a cure. This need not entail any prior or deep commitment: faced with a chronic or life-threatening illness many people will try whatever is available that has been recommended or endorsed by others in the hope that it may prove effective. Many people who use alternative treatments simply have an open mind about what might work. Coupled with dissatisfaction about the quality of care in conventional medicine and its limited efficacy for many chronic illnesses, this openness is sufficient motivation to explore alternatives. As well, people may use some forms of CAM because they are less costly than conventional medical treatments, which remain economically out of reach (Pagan and Pauly 2005).

Pathologies of Reason?

Writing from the perspective of a biomedical practitioner, in a journal for medical education, Beyerstein (2001) has detailed some of the social and psychological reasons for the widespread support of scientifically unproven and implausible complementary and alternative medicine. Among the social reasons he lists are poor scientific literacy and anti-intellectualism or anti-scientism. By poor scientific literacy, Beyerstein means a lack of knowledge of science, or, more specifically, enough background knowledge to be able to read, understand, and minimally evaluate scientific information. This includes not only a technical vocabulary, conceptual models, and familiarity with a style of argument, but also certain epistemological attitudes and social values. Given that most people have neither the time nor the inclination to think through the rationale for technical decisions, but rely instead on the opinion of experts, scientific literacy is often less a matter of reading and reasoning than it is a matter of trust in or deference to a specific type of authority.

While biomedical practitioners are trained to look for the evidence that supports a novel treatment to make "rational" choices of therapy, most people have not acquired the background knowledge needed to see how a treatment fits into a larger picture of the body as a biophysical machine, nor do they necessarily subscribe to this form of scientific materialism. For physicians who draw their professional authority and credibility, as well as their self-confidence, from working within the biomedical model, the mere fact that a treatment does not have a ready biological rationale makes it suspect.[4]

Beyerstein sees anti-intellectualism and anti-scientific attitudes as supported by "New Age mysticism." This New Age mysticism may include an uncritical acceptance of non-Western medicines as rooted in spiritual traditions (for example, the simplistic assumption that Chinese medicine is directly based on Taoism or Ayurveda on Hinduism). However, many people embrace complementary medicine not through any affinity for New Age rhetoric but because certain practices fit with or are integral to their religious values or spiritual aspirations. The use of prayer in healing, for example, is supported by people from diverse backgrounds (including physicians), most of whom do not see themselves as "New Age mystics," but may be Christians or belong to other traditions and ground their healing practices in their religious convictions (Schneirov and Gczik 2004).[5] Insofar as both Christians and celebrants of the New Age situate their use of alternative medicine in larger systems of belief, what these have in common is an ontology that credits the existence of a vital energy or spiritual forces that can affect health.

This ontology is viable, in an age of scientific rationality, for several reasons. Although some proponents of alternative medicine hope for scientific confirmation of its efficacy, they remain insulated from empirical refutation. Faced with contradictory evidence from observation or experiment, they can always appeal to extenuating circumstances, auxiliary hypotheses, or else jump ship, abandoning the scientific paradigm altogether.[6] This reluctance to accept science as the final arbiter of truth is not a lapse in rationality but a continuation of the pragmatic coordination of knowledge as a patchwork quilt of different domains and modes of authority that has characterized most practical reason. As Ernest Gellner argued, for most of history, limited, local, domain-restricted forms of empiricism have been sufficient for most everyday purposes (Gellner 1988). The demand that knowledge be reconciled across widely disparate domains, which is characteristic of modernity, is still not accepted by most people, who comfortably live with segmented systems of practical knowledge deployed for specific purposes.

Metaphor, Embodiment, and Conviction

Another mode of reasoning, characteristic of New Age writing, but actually more pervasive, is the appeal to "intuitive" ways of knowing that are grounded in bodily, emotional, and "spiritual" experiences. These experiences may be intense and compelling, and resist being "explained away" as meaningless or merely a glitch in one's (physiological) system, the result of expectancy or suggestion, misperception, or misinterpretation. The salience, sensory primacy, and obdurate quality of bodily experience warrants the reality of more abstract metaphysical notions. Entire systems of medical knowledge may be built on the correlations of specific actions (eating certain foods) and bodily responses (Nichter 2008).

The cognitive theory of metaphor can shed much light on ways of thinking in traditional medicine and other systems of knowledge (Kirmayer 1992, 2004; Slingerland 2008). The metaphoric extension of bodily experiences stands at the base of our more abstract cognitive constructions (Lakoff and Johnson 1980; Johnson 1987). These metaphoric implications are not entirely supplanted by abstract meanings but continue to exert a constant tug on our ways of thinking. The sensory and emotional connotations of metaphors contribute to our everyday understanding and response to all forms of language, whether spoken or written text, no matter how abstract. There is a psychophysiology of metaphor in which the bodily responses evoked by words contribute to their meaning, both over time as metaphorical meanings are sedimented in the etymology of words, and in the moment as metaphoric connotations evoke physical responses (Gibbs 2006; Barsalou 2008; Geary 2011).

In explaining these modes of thinking in terms of metaphor, we are adopting an *emic* stance, describing the logic and tropic structures of illness and healing from outside the ontological frameworks of the tradition. The cognitive psychological, affective, and rhetorical functions of metaphor can account for much of the efficacy of ritual healing. However, for participants within the tradition, spirits, forces, and energies are not metaphors for anything but primary constituents of all experience, the real essences or presences behind the events we observe. Within the ontology of an ethnomedical system, the energies, qualities of hot or cold, or other features that can be construed metaphorically are seen as literal properties, essences, or motive forces that animate and explain the logic of medicine and healing efficacy. In Hindu forms of worship, for example, statues and other ritual accoutrements are not "symbolic" of deity but actually incorporate it, according to indigenous theories. Ritual healing, then, is not a metaphoric means to a psychological end but a kind of embodied action with direct effects on the spiritual and moral order (Bourdieu 1998; Sax 2009; Quack 2010). There is no inferential process or effort to believe but simply a tacit acceptance—though, to varying degrees, people can be led to ponder and doubt their reality, whether through unexpected failures or encounters with alternative worldviews.

The tendency to literalize or concretize metaphor, for which Paracelsus was criticized, is not simply a matter of careless, imprecise, or impressionistic use of language, but in the nature of embodied knowing (Gibbs 2006; Slingerland 2008). The experience of excitement, edginess, and arousal is naturally metaphorized as "energy," and energy, in turn, hypostatized as something contained and quantifiable in the body or the cosmos. So systems of medicine based on the balance of "energies" can claim not only an internal structural coherence but also a palpable presence in the phenomenology of everyday experience. Energy then becomes not a traveling metaphor but something as phenomenologically real, immediate, and insistent as the experience of excitement itself and, when made central to an elaborate system of correspondences and explanations set down in medical texts, potentially more real than the largely hidden world that biomedicine takes for its reality, which often contradicts everyday experience.[7]

Transcending the Limits of Biomedicine

Behind the enthusiasm for complementary medicine is a growing dissatisfaction with contemporary medicine and a distrust of medical authority, which is increasingly viewed as self-serving or as in the pocket of the pharmaceutical industry.[8] Critiques of Western medicine for its narrow views of efficacy and outcome and its obvious conflicts of interest motivate the search for alternative forms of healing. More trenchantly, biomedicine has been criticized for its failure to engage the personal and cultural dimensions of suffering.

Contemporary biomedicine has adopted an essentialized view of human suffering that focuses primarily on the disease rather than the suffering person and his or her illness. Patients are synonymous with their diagnosis or damaged organ ("the diabetic," "the kidney in bed three") and clinicians aim to treat the disease rather than the patient. When patients' symptoms and experiences of illness do not follow the prototype of a disease found in medical textbooks, they are viewed as "difficult," and the reality of their suffering is suspect. A dualistic ontology distinguishes between real disease and imaginary illnesses, the latter including hypochondriasis, but also other psychological conditions in which people are somehow held responsible for their own conditions. In the case of biomedicine, the textbook representation of disease is so strong that the text occludes the person, thus making for a very alienating experience: patients who report symptoms that do not fit the model of the disease they are presumed to have may be viewed as malingering, histrionic, hysterical, or simply "poor historians"—their story is incoherent because it does not fit the narrative templates in the textbook (Kirmayer 1988, 2000). This split between biologically grounded, real disease and self-induced or fabricated illness, for which the person is ultimately responsible, can be found even among psychiatrists committed to an integrative view of illness (Kirmayer 2000; Miresco and Kirmayer 2006).

Although drawing from diverse medical systems and traditions, each of the many systems grouped together under the rubric of CAM produce their own root metaphors and evocative language that reflect the local contexts of reception as well as global marketing strategies. In France and Québec, alternative medicine has been referred to as *"médecine douce,"* soft medicine, with connotations of being mild or gentle. The metaphorical connotations of CAMs are part of their persuasive appeal, as people reason analogically from the "gentle," harmonious, balanced qualities ascribed to the healing intervention to the desired transformations of experience (Kaptchuk and Eisenberg 1998). Of course, the metaphorical connotations of healing practices may enhance or detract from their efficacy. As much as CAM is viewed in positive terms, reinforced by practices that may involve sensory experiences that are pleasurable or intriguing, biomedicine may involve painful, disorienting, and disturbing treatments aimed not at comfort but biological efficacy. The hospital environment is full of unpleasant sights, sounds, and smells, and the effect may be harsh, frightening, and dispiriting. In contrast, in North America, practitioners of CAM typically invoke notions of nature, wholeness, and harmony that are reassuring, and interventions may be delivered in pleasant surroundings that evoke feelings of safety, comfort, and well-being. In other settings, different sensory associations may be evoked that have associations with power and efficacy (Hinton, Howes, and Kirmayer 2008; Nichter 2008).

There is a substantial mystification in the use of the words "natural" and "holistic" in discussions of CAM.[9] The term "natural" has connotations of gentle, balanced, and harmonious, evoking a return to a mode of experience before artifice and industry. Natural is contrasted with artificial, manufactured, and "chemical," all of which imply human interference. In fact, of course, remedies labeled "natural" usually involve highly complex and largely unknown mixtures of chemicals that vary widely from one batch, branch, or leaf to the next. But the prodigious complexity of nature and its obvious indifference to human need is not enough to undermine the comforting resonance of the term "natural." The "natural" conjures a selective view of nature, defanged, tamed, and comfortable. Nature, then, is the utopian place from which we are estranged in illness and to which we wish to return. In its pristine form, nature is untouched by human hands and contains all that is healthy, whole, and complete (Herzlich and Graham 1973). It is as though something precious is lost in the act of purification and packaging, or that some taint of the ills of urbanization and industrialization are conferred on medication through its manufacture.

"Holistic" implies a comprehensive, integrative approach to illness that includes body, mind, social context, and spirit. However, the interventions of holistic medicine are often manifestly somatic or physical: taking herbal remedies or undergoing the physical manipulations of acupuncture, massage, moxibustion, and chiropractic. On the face of it, such physical treatments are no more holistic than most biomedical remedies. However, the rationale for these somatic interventions uses metaphors of energy, balance, harmony, and spirituality that invoke metaphysical notions that go well beyond the materialist framework of biomedicine. It is this alternative metaphysics that imbues even purely physical interventions with other levels of symbolic meaning. Much of the talk that surrounds holistic treatment is couched in terms of processes that refer to these metaphysical assumptions. At the same time, the use of metaphors like energy, which has a simple correspondence to bodily experiences of vitality, arousal, and emotional activation, gives an experiential grounding and empirical reality to the metaphysical system.

Interestingly, many forms of CAM and traditional medicine (including Indian Ayurveda and traditional Chinese medicine) track symptoms closely, and treatment is adjusted in an ongoing way in response to changes in symptomatology. This close tracking and response to changes in symptoms is likely one very important reason for the perception that CAM is more sensitive to patients' needs and, hence, more holistic. Although in the West, CAM practitioners may offer their patients longer visits, in many South Asian settings, patients have little opportunity to present their story to traditional healers and are simply told what to do by the healer. Nevertheless, the fact that in such systems of medicine patients' symptom experiences often are tracked may contribute to the sense that, even in these settings, some traditional practitioners are perceived as more open, attentive, and responsive than biomedical physicians to their patients' needs and concerns. This tracking of experience is also one way the metaphoric logic of CAM is stabilized as people are taught to reframe and reinterpret their bodily experiences in ways that confirm the explanatory power of the system.

A Medicine of the Imagination

The arena in contemporary biomedicine where some vestige of the Renaissance respect for the imagination can still be found is the clinical and research tradition of psychosomatic medicine. Psychosomatic medicine positions itself somewhere between the extremes of skepticism and credulity: neither so credulous as to adopt the sort of psychological omnipotence that assumes that any illness can be cured by simply wishing it so, nor so skeptical or reductionistic to insist that only simple physiological processes can explain disease and healing (Pressman 1998; Mizrachi 2001; Lipsitt 2006).[10] Psychosomatics searches for the chain of material causes that stretch all the way from healing words, thoughts, images, and emotions to changes in bodily processes. In this quest for causal explanation, observational and experimental methods of science have shown how the exercise of the faculties of imagination can have healing efficacy, bridging the ontological divide of mind and body. Many different processes may contribute to this efficacy, including changes in expectations, coping, and the interpretation of experience, and in interpersonal interaction, as well as physiology (Kirmayer 2003, 2004).

There is a good deal of evidence that expectations of therapeutic effects lead to both cognitive and physiological changes (Kirsch 1999). This family of diverse responses has been called the placebo effect, but there are really many different effects, depending on the bodily systems and psychological responses activated (Benedetti 2009). In addition to conscious expectations, many different symbolic aspects of a placebo may elicit a response, including its appearance and other sensory qualities. Moerman (2002) has argued that the placebo effect might be better named the "meaning effect," since the outcome depends on the meanings ascribed to the stimulus. However, this is meaning in a very extended sense because some of the symbolic effects of the placebo may be at the level of sensory cues or associations, or even unconditioned responses that require little cognitive mediation. Thus, the meanings mobilized through placebos are embodied as well as metaphoric and metonymic (Kirmayer 2011). It is not only the explicit story, narrative fragment, or prediction—"This medicine is effective, therefore you will get better"—that may be effective, but also specific evocative meanings and connotations: "This pill has essential nutrients. It will nourish you and make you stronger." Indeed, this message of strengthening and subsequent feelings of getting stronger may be enacted, experienced, and expressed in ways that are not encoded or mediated in words but in bodily gestures and sensorimotor processes.

The evocative power of specific sounds, words, phrases, and longer narratives or stories stems both from their intrinsic metaphoricity and their developmental history. Some of this is shared cultural history and some will be idiosyncratic to any individual; hence each person's pattern of response to specific stimuli will be unique. The same goes for the conditioned effects that contribute to placebo responses. They depend on the learning history of the individual, which has forged links between specific stimuli and responses. This makes research studies that lump together groups of people with disparate learning histories a poor method for showing the impact of symbolic meaning: the same event may mean quite different things to different people and elicit different psychophysiological responses. Some of this response is simple associative learning with little cognitive mediation, but much involves more complex interpretations of the significance of events based on knowledge and active construction of meaning.

Healing can be understood as a process of metaphorical transformation in which representations of the self are mapped onto the realms created by imaginative models and overarching myths in ways that transform the experiential qualities and meaning of self as body and psyche (Kirmayer 2003, 2004). These representational realms or spaces acquire their depth or multiple layers through developmental experiences so that metaphoric transformations affect not only specific denotations of words but also connotative levels of meaning involving emotional, sensory, and gestural qualities. Language then gains a psychophysiological effectiveness that works hand in hand with its rhetorical power.

Ritual action and narration may heal by allowing symbolic closure, bringing a sense of formal completeness or coherent emplotment to the fragmented and chaotic elements of illness experience (Herzfeld 1986; Mattingly 1994). It may transform the meaning of experience by conferring metaphorical qualities or blending representational spaces (Sweetser 2000). It may build solidarity with others through shared accounts of suffering in socially understandable and valorized terms (Kirmayer 2000; Sax 2009). Finally, narration may open up new possibilities, subjunctivizing predicaments viewed as fixed and unchangeable (Good 1994). The healing efficacy of words, then, can be attributed to multiple levels of effect: to creating positive expectations, either in terms of general hopefulness or more specific expectations for change; to forging supportive and comforting relationships with others; and through the sense that one is not alone and that one's suffering has meaning for oneself and others.

Contemporary psychosomatic medicine provides ample evidence of causal interactions between psychological and somatic processes (Blumenfield and Strain 2006). Given the scientific evidence for an integrative view of illness causation and healing, it is striking how much dualistic thinking persists in the clinical reasoning of psychiatrists and other biomedical practitioners (Miresco and Kirmayer 2006). Some illnesses are viewed as predominately biological in causation and others as psychological. Psychological conditions are more likely to be seen as due to the individual's actions and hence to be associated with moral blame. This is one of the roots of the persistent stigma attached to mental illness.

The Persistence of Dualism

The idea of mind-body medicine aims to address a dualism that is deeply rooted in Western tradition. However, some of the distinctions found in mind-body dualism are not confined to any particular tradition but emerge from the phenomenology of experience (Kirmayer 1988; Lambek 1998). The contrast between the limitlessness of imagination and the finitude of bodily life is likely an existential universal. Of course, particular configurations of this contrast reflect culture-specific ontologies and corresponding notions of the person (Ozawa de-Silva 2002; Ozawa de-Silva and Ozawa de-Silva 2011; Shulman, 2012). These notions of the person and the larger cosmologies in which they are situated give rise to different systems of healing.

In this era of globalization, a great variety of forms of healing are readily available to people from diverse backgrounds. However, the degree of use of a particular type of healing need not correlate with individuals' understanding of or commitment to its associated ontology. The extent to which individuals are expected or need to engage with the ontology (either experientially or in terms of theory or metaphysics) varies with the healing system, setting, and practitioner. Specifically, it depends on how the healing system makes use of metaphors, interpretive frameworks, epistemologies that are explicitly tied to the ontology. For example "energy" may be deployed as an abstract concept that allows analogical mapping across different systems, as an experiential index of healing activity or efficacy, or as a clinical phenomenon that requires learning to attend to (or imagine) specific sensations. The different versions of energy in diverse healing systems are only superficially analogous; the meaning system in which *ki* or *chi* is embedded differs from that of the energies, "winds," "humors," or powers recognized by other traditions. And, of course, none of these notions of energy or healing power has any close correspondence to the technical meaning of energy in biomedicine (which is based on the physical chemistry of the molecular machinery of the cell). To clarify the points of commonality and divergence in the cultural elaboration of metaphoric meaning, we can distinguish several levels of potential correspondence across healing systems: embodied experience; indexes; metaphoric connotations; denotative meaning related to their location in an ethnomedical system; and relationships to explicit ontologies.

Metaphoric universals may undergird the structure of humoral systems of medicine, from the simplest hot/cold system to the elaborate structures of Ayurveda. While the elaborate systems of literate traditions of medicine have more complex narrative structures, in practice they are often delivered either with a blunt expression of authority or a metaphoric argument that appeals directly to bodily sensations and intuitions. The global marketing of traditional medicines then involves a thinning out of the social and cultural embedding of interventions, a repackaging and re-presentation of key metaphors that relies on the interplay between embodied experience and the circulation of popular ideologies of health for their plausibility and acceptance (Kirmayer 2008).

44

If we take seriously the great cultural diversity of forms of healing found around the world, we can either assume that everything works the same way—creating positive expectations, remoralizing the person, integrating the self, or balancing "energy"—or notice that diverse processes are involved. The interest in mind-body medicine is not just empirically to establish efficacy and effectiveness more rigorously, but also to work out the mechanisms so that we have a sound basis for deciding where to turn in any given instance. All of the levels of potential effectiveness of any healing practice need not be accounted for within its own explanatory system. The claims of efficacy of any system must be examined critically because there are many reasons why both patients and practitioners might, consciously or unintentionally, overstate the case.

Healing involves basic bodily processes of balancing, homeostatic regulation, and repair, but it is equally a matter of making sense of suffering and finding a way to carry on. The parallel semiotics of body and text presents us with another fundamental doubling, one that is not dualistic or dichotomous but multilayered, cooperative, and synergistic (Kirmayer 1992). All forms of healing share in common the potential to modify experience at multiple levels through the psychophysiology of metaphor, the structuring of narrative, and the social dynamics of rhetoric. The experience of word magic, based on the power of words to conjure and transform reality, lies behind our more self-conscious and critical uses of language to argue, clarify, and describe. Words may be used in many different ways to heal: through magical invocation, supplication, or prayer; through dialogue that brings one person into relation with an other, present or imagined; as recipes to follow, sources of instructions and imperatives; as conceptual toolkits, sources of metaphors, analogies, and models to think with; as instruments to focus and occupy consciousness, as in the use of mantras; as objects of aesthetic contemplation, as in lyric poetry, to admire their sound and fit; and as stories to dwell within or labyrinths to explore. Each of these has associated with it ways of inhabiting the body and transforming consciousness. Becoming aware of the ways that language shapes experience does not dissolve its transformative effects but it affords us new opportunities for situated understanding and critique of our own beliefs and convictions.

Belief, faith, and conviction about the effectiveness of diverse forms of healing also rest on links with other aspects of individual and collective identity, including religion, ethnicity, and language. Use of particular healing practices then becomes not only a search for cure, but also a process of strengthening personal, professional, or collective identities and elaborating ethical positions and commitments. This, as much as the hope for cure, and the economic stakes, accounts for the intensity with which healing practices may be held, challenged, and defended.

Conclusion: Pluralism and the Ideologies of Health and Healing

We live in a global agora where diverse forms of medicine coexist and compete for attention, credibility, and resources. In this contest, the local orthodoxies of "traditional" or indigenous medicines risk becoming marginalized unless they adopt the rhetoric, packaging, and marketing of the economic mainstream. As traditional forms of medicine circulate internationally they are redefined against the backdrop of biomedicine and thrown together as "complementary and alternative." Practitioners and clients are impelled to accept this redefinition because of the promise of a measure of legitimacy and access to wider markets. In so doing, however, the overt challenge that alternative systems of medicine present to biomedicine may be muted since all appear to be speaking the same language of efficacy and efficiency. But because they are rooted in fundamentally different ontologies, important tensions and contradictions remain. These different ontologies are attractive to some because they appear to bridge the divide between mind and body that continues to pose dilemmas for patients and healers in biomedicine.

Traditional healing practices were deeply rooted in a whole worldview, built up over the course of an individual's life through developmental experiences that gave the symbols of healing their evocative power and resonance. In a globalizing world, people have ready access to many forms of medicine that have no deep roots in their own traditions or experience. Instead, these forms of medicine come wrapped in the packaging of global marketing strategies with only cursory adaptations to local idioms. The question that arises is whether the efficacy of such imported interventions is the same as when these are delivered within the cultural contexts from which they emerged. What social underpinning, cultural background knowledge, or experience is needed to make a form of healing efficacious?

To realize the benefit of a healing system, it must have some credibility and sustainability over time, both as a practice to which one can return repeatedly and as a discursive system that is valorized and reinforced in the larger social world. Healing does not occur just in the moment of ritualized encounter or treatment but in the subsequent lived contexts in which new ways of understanding and inhabiting the body are practiced, both alone and with others. Healing practices can extend, enhance or confer new identities in ways that may have private meaning for the sufferer's self-understanding and autobiography. To have the greatest impact, however, these identities must be deployed in the wider social world where they become part of larger ideologies that serve not only to sustain the institutions of health care but also to explain and maintain the central institutions of global society. The result is a pluralistic medical system in which the marketplace elides fundamental differences in ontology under a hegemonic view of health and healing consistent with neoliberal definitions of the person as a consumer actively engaged with health services to further the projects of self-fashioning and self-care.

Acknowledgments

Portions of this chapter are adapted with permission from: Kirmayer, Laurence J. 2006. "Toward a Medicine of the Imagination." *New Literary History* 37(3): 583–605. I thank William S. Sax, Johannes Quack, the anonymous reviewers, and members of the Therapy in Translation working group, Minerva Center for Humanities, Tel Aviv University, for helpful comments on earlier drafts.

Notes

1. There is a dualism in Plato that becomes a trialism in Aristotle of body/soul/ spirit (Fortenbaugh 1975). This is reflected, for example, in the psychophysiology of medieval Jewish mysticism, which distinguishes three parts or aspects of the soul: *ruach*, *nefesh*, and *neshamah* (self, spirit, and breath) (Kottek 1979).
2. However, there is no simple opposition between CAM and conventional medicine, since a growing number of biomedical practitioners also refer patients to CAM or offer certain modalities themselves (Wiese, Oster, and

Pincombe 2010). In 2000, about 40 percent of general practitioners in the U.K. offered access to CAM, most commonly, referring patients to chiropractors or osteopaths for the treatment of chronic low back pain (A. Vickers 2000). In Israel, complementary medicine has been integrated into multimodal primary care clinics, in part to attract and retain patients in a competitive environment, but this is no guarantee of satisfaction with services (Fadlon 2004; Shuval and Mizrachi 2004; Mizrachi, Shuval, and Gross 2005). Indeed, the adoption of CAM by biomedical practitioners provides a measure of legitimation that may benefit nonbiomedical practitioners, who nevertheless remain ambivalent about this appropriation of their territory (Wiese and Oster 2010).

3. Clinical researchers distinguish between *efficacy,* the ability of a treatment to cause a positive outcome under ideal circumstances (e.g., with a selected sample under laboratory conditions), and *effectiveness,* the actual impact of a treatment in a real-world context.

4. The limitations of everyday clinical reasoning have spurred the recent movement for evidence-based medicine, which aims to get physicians to follow rational treatment guidelines founded on the weight of empirical evidence (Whitley, Rousseau, Carpenter-Song, and Kirmayer 2011). However, the production of scientific evidence is costly and, in many areas, slow to accrue. As a result, many common treatments remain untested and many specific clinical questions unanswered. Even where good evidence on treatment efficacy is available, it is couched in terms of probabilities based on populations that may not match the individual before the clinician. There is always the additional challenge of translating the generic knowledge produced by scientific research into appropriate interventions for a specific individual. This leaves open a lot of room for physicians to incorporate alternative treatments without undermining the conceptual edifice or scientific commitments of biomedicine. So we must consider broader cultural issues to understand the resistance to CAM within biomedicine, as well as its embrace by large segments of the general population.

5. Indeed, from mid century until the 1960s, alternative medicine in the United States was largely the province of the Christian right, associated with mistrust of secular institutions and anti-Semitism (see Collins and Pinch 2005).

6. For example, in response to a randomized clinical trial of intercessory prayer for people undergoing cardiac bypass operations, which found no benefit, physician Harold Koenig, director of the Center for Spirituality, Theology and Health at the Duke University Medical Center, commented, "Science is not designed to study the supernatural" (Ritter 2006). Yet, Koenig has been a prominent advocate of scientific research on the impact of religiosity and spirituality on health and healing (Koenig 2009).

7. Interestingly, there is evidence that there is an economy of cognitive effort that underlies experiences of "energy" and performance and this can be linked to actual metabolic processes in specific brain systems. For example,

blood glucose levels are related to the capacity to exert "willpower" or self-control (Gailliot et al. 2007). But the detailed correspondences between experience, performance, and brain activity are far more complex than the broad use of the "energy" metaphors in the discourse of CAM.

8. Alternative practitioners are sometimes portrayed as less motivated than biomedical physicians by commercial interests. Yet they must compete for clients and market their skills. A newspaper article described research on the beneficial effects of omega-3 fatty acids (found in fish oil) and quoted psychiatrist David Servan-Schreiber to the effect that, unlike the situation with antidepressant medications, no pharmaceutical company had a vested interest in promoting fish oil or inflating its claims for efficacy: "But you can't patent fish oil," Servan-Schreiber said when asked why alternative methods have been given little attention. "No one has an economic interest in making them widely available" (Fidelman 2006). In fact, the omega-3 market was valued at $195 million in 2004 and was expected to grow at an average annual rate of 8 percent. Dr. Servan-Schreiber was the author of a popular book on healing that promoted fish oil (*The Instinct to Heal: Curing Stress, Anxiety, and Depression without Drugs and without Talk Therapy*, Servan-Schreiber, 2004) and consultant to a company that sold omega-3 dietary supplements. His website, www.guerir.fr ("heal stress, anxiety and depression without medications or psychoanalysis") offered a checklist of common somatic symptoms of stress and encourages readers to explore treatments including relaxation training, physical exercise, EMDR (Eye Movement Desensitization and Reprocessing, a therapy for trauma-related disorders), bright light therapy, acupuncture, emotional communication, and the use of omega-3 supplements.

9. The notion of holism has had multiple meanings in the history of medicine and is associated not only with integrative thinking but with institutional issues related to the medical profession and the emergence of medical specialties (cf. Lawrence and Weisz 1998).

10. On the fantasy of omnipotence, see Seidenberg (1963). On the other hand, psychosomatic medicine still needs defending from arch reductionists who believe that psychological attitudes count for little in the face of the powerful biological processes of disease (see Williams, Schneiderman, Relman, and Angell 2002).

References

Andrews, Gavin J., Jon Adams, and Jeremy Segrott. 2009. "Complementary and Alternative Medicine (CAM): Production, Consumption, Research." In *A Companion to Health and Medical Geography*, ed. Tim Brown, Sara McLafferty, and Graham Moon. Oxford, U.K.: Blackwell, 587–603.

Barnes, Patricia M., Eve Powell-Griner, Kim McFann, and Richard L. Nahin. 2004. "Complementary and Alternative Medicine Use Among Adults: United States, 2002." *Seminars in Integrative Medicine*, 2(2): 54-71.

Barsalou, Lawrence W. 2008. "Grounded Cognition." *Annual Review of Psychology*, 59: 617–645.

Benedetti, Fabrizio. 2009. *Placebo Effects: Understanding the Mechanisms in Health and Disease*. Oxford: Oxford University Press.

Beyerstein, Barry L. 2001. "Alternative Medicine and Common Errors of Reasoning." *Academic Medicine* 76(3): 230–237.

Blumenfield, Michael, and James J. Strain. 2006. *Psychosomatic Medicine*. Philadelphia: Lippincott Williams & Wilkins.

Bourdieu, Pierre. 1998. *Practical Reason: On the Theory of Action*. Stanford: Stanford University Press.

Carey, Benedict. 2006. "When Trust in Doctors Erodes, Other Treatments fill the Void." *New York Times*. February 3.

Chaves, Mark. 2010. "Rain Dances in the Dry Season: Overcoming the Religious Congruence Fallacy." *Journal for the Scientific Study of Religion* 49: 1–14.

Claus, David B. 1981. *Toward the Soul: An Inquiry into the Meaning of Psyche before Plato*. New Haven: Yale University Press.

Collins, Harry, and Trevor Pinch. 2005. *Dr. Golem: How to Think about Medicine*. Chicago: University of Chicago Press.

Daniel, E. Valentine. 1984. *Fluid Signs: Being a Person the Tamil Way*. Berkeley: University of California Press.

Darnton, Robert. 1968. *Mesmerism and the End of the Enlightenment in France*. New York: Schocken Books.

Daston, Lorraine. 1998. "Fear and Loathing of the Imagination in Science." *Daedalus* 127: 73–96.

Doniger, Wendy. 1997. "Medical and Mythical Constructions of the Body in Hindu Texts." In *Religion and the Body*. ed. Sarah Coakley. New York: Cambridge University Press, 167–184 .

Ellenberger, Henri F. 1970. *The Discovery of the Unconscious: The History and Evolution of Dynamic Psychiatry*. New York: Basic Books.

Ernst, Waltraud. 2004. "Colonial Psychiatry, Magic and Religion: The Case of Mesmerism in British India." *History of Psychiatry* 15(1): 57–71.

———. 2007. "Beyond East and West: From the History of Colonial Medicine to a Social History of Medicine(s) in South Asia." *Social History of Medicine* 20(3): 505–524.

Fadlon, Judith. 2004. "Unrest in Utopia: Israeli Patients' Dissatisfaction with Non-conventional Medicine." *Social Science and Medicine* 58(12): 2421–2429.

Fidelman, C. 2006. "Lifting Depression the Natural Way." *The Gazette (Montreal)*. January 12.

Fischer-Homberger, Esther. 1979. "On the Medical History of the Doctrine of Imagination." *Psychological Medicine* 9(4): 619–628.

Fortenbaugh, William W. 1975. *Aristotle on Emotion: A Contribution to Philosophical Psychology, Rhetoric, Poetics, Politics and Ethics*. London: Duckworth.

Foucault, Michel. 1994. *The Birth of the Clinic: An Archaeology of Medical Perception*. New York: Vintage Books.

Fuller, Robert C. 1982. *Mesmerism and the American Cure of Souls*. Philadelphia: University of Pennsylvania Press.

Gailliot, Matthew T., Baumeister Roy F., Nathan DeWall, Jon K. Maner, E. Ashby Plant, Dianne M. Tice, Lauren E. Brewer, and Brandon J. Schmeichel. 2007. "Self-control Relies on Glucose as a Limited Energy Source: Willpower is More than a Metaphor." *Journal of Personality and Social Psychology* 92(2): 325–336.

Gauld, Alan. 1992. *A History of Hypnotism*. New York: Cambridge University Press.

Geary, James. 2011. *I is an Other*. New York: Harper.

Gellner, Ernest. 1988. *Plough, Sword and Book: The Structure of Human History*. Chicago: University of Chicago Press.

Gibbs, Raymond W. 2006. *Embodiment and Cognitive Science*. New York: Cambridge University Press.

Good, Byron J. 1994. *Medicine, Rationality, and Experience: An Anthropological Perspective*. Cambridge: Cambridge University Press.

Herzfeld, M. 1986. "Closure as Cure: Tropes in the Exploration of Bodily and Social Disorder." *Current Anthropology* 27(2): 107–112.

Herzlich, C., and D. Graham. 1973. *Health and Illness*. London: Academic Press.

Hilgard, Josephine R. 1979. *Personality and Hypnosis: A Study of Imaginative Involvement*. Chicago: University of Chicago Press.

Hinton, Devon E., David Howes, and Laurence J. Kirmayer. 2008. "Toward a Medical Anthropology of Sensations: Definitions and Research Agenda." *Transcultural Psychiatry* 45(2): 142–162.

Jacobi, Jolande. 1988. *Paracelsus: Selected Writings*. Princeton: Princeton University Press.

Johnson, Mark. 1987. *The Body in the Mind: The Bodily Basis of Meaning, Imagination and Reason*. Chicago: University of Chicago Press.

Kahneman, Daniel. 2003. "A Perspective on Judgment and Choice: Mapping Bounded Rationality." *American Psychologist* 58(9): 697–720.

———. 2011. *Thinking, Fast and Slow*. New York: Random House.

Kakar, Sudhir. 1982. *Shamans, Mystics, and Doctors: A Psychological Inquiry into India and its Healing Traditions*. Boston: Beacon Press.

Kaptchuk, Ted J., and David M. Eisenberg. 1998. "The Persuasive Appeal of Alternative Medicine." *Annals of Internal Medicine* 129(12): 1061–1065.

Kirmayer, Laurence J. 1988. "Mind and Body as Metaphors: Hidden Values in Biomedicine." In *Biomedicine Examined*, ed. Margaret Lock and Deborah Gordon. Dordrecht: Kluwer Academic Publishers, 57–94.

———. 1992. "The Body's Insistence on Meaning: Metaphor as Presentation and Representation in Illness Experience." *Medical Anthropology Quarterly* 6(4): 323–346.

———. 1993. "Healing and the Invention of Metaphor: The Effectiveness of Symbols Revisited." *Culture, Medicine and Psychiatry* 17(2) 161–195.

———. 2000. "Broken Narratives: Clinical Encounters and the Poetics of Illness Experience." In *Narrative and the Cultural Construction of Illness and*

Healing, ed. Cheryl Mattingly and Linda C. Garro. Berkeley: University of California Press, 153–180.

———. 2003. "Reflections on Embodiment." In *Social and Cultural Lives of Immune Systems,* ed. James M. Wilce. New York: Routledge, 282–302.

———. 2004. "The Cultural Diversity of Healing: Meaning, Metaphor and Mechanism." *British Medical Bulletin* 69(1): 33–48.

———. 2008. "Culture and the Metaphoric Mediation of Pain." *Transcultural Psychiatry* 45(2): 318–338.

———. 2011. "Unpacking the Placebo Response: Insights from Ethnographic Studies of Healing." *The Journal of Mind-Body Regulation* 1(3): 112–124.

———. 2012. "Cultural Competence and Evidence-based Practice in Mental Health: Epistemic Communities and the Politics of Pluralism." *Social Science and Medicine* 75(2): 249–256.

Kirsch, Irving. 1999. *How Expectancies Shape Experience.* Washington D.C.: American Psychological Association.

Koenig, Harold. G. 2009. "Research on Religion, Spirituality and Mental Health: A Review." *Canadian Journal of Psychiatry* 54(5): 283–291.

Kottek, Samuel S. 1979. "The Seat of the Soul: Contribution to the History of Jewish Medieval Psycho-physiology (6th to 12th Century)." *Clio Medica* 13(3-4): 219–246.

Lakoff, George, and Mark Johnson. 1980. *Metaphors We Live By.* Chicago: University of Chicago Press.

Lambek, Michael. 1998. "Body and Mind in Mind, Body and Mind in Body: Some Anthropological Interventions in a Long Conversation." In *Bodies and Persons: Comparative Perspectives from Africa and Melanesia,* ed. Michael Lambek and Andrew Strathern. Cambridge: Cambridge University Press, 103–126.

Lawrence, Christopher, and Geroge Weisz. 1998. *Greater than the Parts: Holism in Biomedicine, 1920-1950.* New York: Oxford University Press.

Lipsitt, Don R. 2006. "Psychosomatic Medicine: History of a 'New' Specialty." In *Psychosomatic Medicine,* ed. Michael Blumenfield and James J. Strian. Philadelphia: Lippincott Williams & Wilkins, 3–20.

Lyng, Stephen. 2010. "Reflexive Biomedicalization and Laternativ Healing Systems." *Journal of Bioethical Inquiry* 7(1): 53–69.

Lynn, Stephen J., and Judith J. Rhue. 1986. "The Fantasy-prone Person: Hypnosis, Imagination and Creativity." *Journal of Personality and Social Psychology* 51(2): 404–408.

Mattingly, Cheryl. 1994. "The Concept of Therapeutic 'Emplotment.'" *Social Science and Medicine* 38(6): 811–822.

McConkey, Kevin M., and Campbell Perry. 2002. "Benjamin Franklin and Mesmerism, Revisited." *International Journal of Clinical and Experimental Hypnosis* 50(4): 320–331.

Micale, Mark S. 1995. *Approaching Hysteria: Disease and Its Interpretations.* Princeton: Princeton University Press.

Miresco, Mark J., and Laurence J. Kirmayer. 2006. "The Persistence of Mind-brain Dualism in Psychiatric Reasoning about Clinical Scenarios." *American Journal of Psychiatry* 163(5): 913–918.

Mizrachi, Nissim. 2001. "From Causation to Correlation: The Story of Psychosomatic Medicine 1939-1979." *Culture, Medicine and Psychiatry* 25(3): 317–343.

Mizrachi, Nissim, Judith T. Shuval, and Sky Gross. 2005. "Boundary at Work: Alternative Medicine in Biomedical Settings." *Sociology of Health and Illness* 27(1): 20–43.

Moerman, Daniel E. 2002. *Meaning, Medicine and the "Placebo Effect."* New York: Cambridge University Press.

Nguyen, Long T., Roger B. Davis, Ted J. Kaptchuk, and Russell S. Phillips. 2011. "Use of Complementary and Alternative Medicine and Self-rated Health Status: Results from a National Survey." *Journal of General Internal Medicine* 26(4): 399–404.

Nichter, Mark 2008. "Coming to Our Senses: Appreciating the Sensorial in Medical Anthropology." *Transcultural Psychiatry* 45(2): 163–197.

Ozawa-de Silva, Chikako. 2002. "Beyond the Body/Mind? Japanese Contemporary Thinkers on Alternative Sociologies of the Body." *Body & Society* 8(2): 21–38.

Ozawa-de Silva, Chikako, and Brendan R. Ozawa-de Silva, 2011. "Mind/Body Theory and Practice in Tibetan Medicine and Buddhism." *Body & Society* 17(1): 95–119.

Pagan, Jose A., and Mark V. Pauly. 2005. "Access to Conventional Medical Care and the Use of Complementary and Alternative Medicine." *Health Affairs (Millwood)* 24(1): 255–262.

Pagel, Walter. 1982. *Paracelsus: An Introduction to Philosophical Medicine in the Era of the Renaissance.* Basel: Karger.

Pressman, Jack D. 1998. "Human Understanding: Psychosomatic Medicine and the Mission of the Rockefeller Foundation." In *Greater than the Parts: Holism in Biomedicine, 1920-1950,* ed. Christopher Lawrence, and George Weisz. New York: Oxford University Press, 189–207.

Quack, Johannes. 2010. "Bell, Bourdieu and Wittgenstein on Ritual Sense." In *The Problem of Ritual Efficacy,* ed. William S. Sax, Johannes Quack, and Jan Weinhold. Oxford, U.K.: Oxford University Press, 169–188.

Quah, Stella. R. 2003. "Traditional Healing Systems and the Ethos of Science." *Social Science and Medicine* 57(10): 1997–2012.

Ritter, M. 2006. "Healing Power of Prayer Debunked." *The Gazette (Montreal).* March 31.

Sax, William S. 2009. *God of Justice: Ritual Healing and Social Justice in the Central Himalayas.* New York: Oxford University Press.

———. 2010. "Ritual and the Problem of Efficacy." In *The Problem of Ritual Efficacy,* ed. William S. Sax, Johannes Quack, and Jan Weinhold. Oxford, U.K.: Oxford University Press, 3–16.

Schmit, David. 2005. "Re-visioning Antebellum American Psychology: The Dissemination of Mesmerism, 1836-1854." *History of Psychology* 8(4): 403–434.

Schneirov, Matthew, and Jonathan D. Gczik. 2004. "Beyond the Culture Wars: The Politics of Alternative Healing." In *The Politics of Healing: Histories of*

Alternative Medicine in Twentieth Century North America, ed. Robert D. Johnson. New York: Routledge, 245–258.

Seidenberg, Robert. 1963. "Omnipotence, Denial and Psychosomatic Medicine." *Psychosomatic Medicine* 25(1): 31–36.

Servan-Schreiber, David. 2004. *The Instinct to Heal: Curing Stress, Anxiety and Depression without Drugs and without Talk Therapy*. Emmaus: Rodale.

Shulman, David. 2012. *More Than Real: A History of the Imagination in South India*. Cambridge, M.A.: Harvard University Press.

Shuval, Judith T., and Nissim Mizrachi. 2004. "Changing Boundaries: Modes of Coexistence of Alternative and Biomedicine." *Qualitative Health Research* 14(5): 675–690.

Slingerland, Edward. 2008. *What Science Offers the Humanities: Integrating Body and Culture*. New York: Cambridge University Press.

Solmsen, Friedrich. 1983. "Plato and the Concept of the Soul (Psyche): Some Historical Perspectives." *Journal of the History of Ideas* 44(3): 355–367.

Sullivan, Mark. 1986. "In What Sense is Contemporary Medicine Dualistic?" *Culture, Medicine and Psychiatry* 10(4): 331–350.

Sweetser, Eve. 2000. "Blended Spaces and Performativity." *Cognitive Linguistics* 11(3-4): 305–333.

Temkin, Owsei. 1952. "The Elusiveness of Paracelsus." *Bulletin of the History of Medicine* 26(3): 201–217.

Vickers, Andrew. 2000. "Complementary Medicine." *British Medical Journal* 321(7262): 683–686.

Vickers, Brian. 1984. "Analogy versus Identity: The Rejection of Occult Symbolism, 1580-1680." In *Occult and Scientific Mentalities in the Renaissance*, ed. Brian Vickers. Cambridge, U.K.: Cambridge University Press, 95–164.

Vos, Lynn, and Ross Brennan. 2010. "Complementary and Alternative Medicine: Shaping a Marketing Research Agenda." *Marketing Intelligence & Planning* 28(3): 349–364.

Whitley, Robert, Cécile Rousseau, Elizabeth Carpenter-Song, and Laurence J. Kirmayer. 2011. "Evidence-based Medicine: Opportunities and Challenges in a Diverse Society." *Canadian Journal of Psychiatry* 56(9): 514–522.

Whorton, James C. 2004. "From Cultism to CAM: Alternative Medicine in the Twentieth Century." In *The Politics of Healing: Histories of Alternative Medicine in Twentieth Century North America*, ed. Robert D. Johnson. New York: Routledge, 287–306.

Wiese, Mariene, and Candice Oster. 2010. "'Becoming Accepted': The Complementary and Alternative Medicine Practitioners' Response to the Uptake and Practice of Traditional Medicine Therapies by the Mainstream Health Sector." *Health* 14(4): 415–433.

Wiese, Mariene, Candice Oster, and Jan Pincombe. 2010. "Understanding the Emerging Relationship between Complementary Medicine and Mainstream Health Care: A Review of the Literature." *Health* 14(3): 326–342.

Williams, Redford, Neil Schneiderman, Arnold Relman, and Marcia Angel. 2002. "Resolved: Psychosocial Interventions Can Improve Clinical Outcomes in

Organic Disease—Rebuttals and Closing Arguments." *Psychosomatic Medicine* 64(4): 564–567.

Winter, Alison. 1998. *Mesmerized: Powers of Mind in Victorian Britain*. Chicago: University of Chicago Press.

Wujastyk, Dagmar, and Frederich M. Smith. 2008. *Modern and Global Ayurveda: Pluralism and Paradigms*. Albany: State University of New York.

Zaretsky, Eli. 2004. *Secrets of the Soul: A Social and Cultural History of Psychoanalysis*. New York: Alfred A. Knopf.

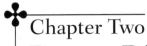

Chapter Two
Porous Dividuals?
Complying to a Healing Temple
(Balaji) and a Psychiatric
Out-Patient Department (OPD)

Johannes Quack

Balaji and OPD:
What Different Institutions Ask For

How many people become possessed by a spirit, deceased relative,
god, or goddess in the out-patient department (OPD) of a psychiatric clinic in India? In the course of my ethnographic research at
a hospital in a North Indian city I neither saw nor heard of such a
case. Patients (and their relatives) did not mention such practices
in front of the doctor, although they did tell me later in interviews
that possession is central to their experience of suffering or to their
help-seeking behavior outside the biomedical realm. The psychiatric setting as I observed it "asks for" behavior that is quite distinct
from possession: patients have to register themselves, pay a small
fee, and wait more or less quietly for their turn. In the clinic in
which I worked they had to bring their old *parcā* (the paper on which
the diagnosis as well as the prescriptions are written) along with
any further documentation of previous treatments, tests, and medication, as no records are kept by the psychiatrist, or the hospital.
In the OPD they have to respect the authority of the doctor and
are supposed to answer the questions of the psychiatrists quickly,
precisely, and without further ado, even if they are unfamiliar with
such questions. Afterward they are expected to buy the prescribed

56

medicine, take the tablets regularly and on time, and return to the clinic, usually every two weeks. If they are willing and able to "comply" by following these demands, the psychiatrist is happy, friendly, and constructive, and the chances of a successful treatment are supposed to be much greater.[1]

In contrast to this, many "patients" (and their relatives) visit healing shrines and temples or local healers and oracles where they may become possessed before, after, or alongside their treatment with the psychiatrist. Balaji healing temple, a North Indian healing and pilgrimage site, is one of the most famous of such places in India. Located just a few kilometers from the main road between Delhi and Jaipur in an otherwise nondescript village called Mehndipur, Balaji draws pilgrims from all over India and even abroad, as well as researchers from all over the world.[2] The place is famous for its healing powers, especially for problems that outsiders, using categories largely absent from the local perspectives, refer to as "psychological" or as signs of "mental illness."[3] The practices that take place there have been well described by a number of scholars from a range of disciplines.[4] I visited Balaji in October 2006 to conduct joint research with anthropologist William Sax and psychologist Jan Weinhold.

The central deity of the temple is Balaji, the child form of the monkey-god Hanuman. The healing deity is well known to everybody, Hanuman being a paradigmatic helper venerated all over India, and in this case accompanied by the "king of ghosts" Pretraj, along with a further set of other local demons and spirits.[5] Besides Balaji, his helpers and temples of the Hindu gods Ram and Shiva and their priests, there are also healing specialists from near and far who deal with the problems of the visitors to Balaji.[6] The way in which help seekers approach Balaji and his helpers resembles that of a court procedure. At first they "file their case" by making one smaller and one larger offering at the main temple. This is referred by using the Urdu legal terms *darkhast* and *arzi*. Second, they obtain a "court hearing" (*peśī*) and in successful cases there is a final "trial," in which Balaji acts as judge and during which the afflicting spirits are usually condemned and sentenced.

Below I focus only on *peśī*, since it is at this stage that dramatic possession takes place, mostly during the *āratī* ceremonies[7] in the morning and evening, or during the day at the *samādhi-sthal*. The *samādhi-sthal* is a space roughly the size of two football fields, with a small temple in the middle that functions as a commemorative shrine (*samādhi*) of the former chief priest (*mahaṃt*) of the temple, Ganeshpuri (1899–1972), who is said to have initiated the distinctive healing practices associated with Balaji. Our research team spent most of its time walking around this space, watching and listening to different forms of consultation and treatment (it is so popular that often several possessions and treatments take place at the same time) or talking to the people about Balaji, their reasons for coming, their experiences, etc. While this gave us an eclectic overview of the various practices taking place, we were also able to observe one case at length, that of a young man in his mid twenties called Sanjay (a pseudonym) who was visiting Balaji with his father. The information we collected on Sanjay was summarized by Sax and Weinhold as follows:

> The father was an ex-soldier who had been able, several years earlier, to get over his drinking problem with the help of Balaji. Since then he had become a regular visitor to the temple, and was representative of a certain type of person for whom the paradigm of spirit possession and the healing power of Balaji become central orienting principles. This man had brought his son Sanjay to the temple for a visit, and soon after his arrival the young man began to exhibit signs of possession. He told us that he had never experienced any particular troubles or difficulties while at home, and that the symptoms of possession appeared only after he came to Balaji. He offered *arzi* and *darkhast*, and soon he could be seen several times a day at the *samādhi-sthal* along with a group of fellow-villagers from Haryana, exhibiting typical signs of possession: shaking and trembling, kneeling on the ground, rotating his head rapidly, and the like. This was *peśī*, and it was positively regarded, since it indicated that Balaji was actively seeking to drive out the afflicting spirit. While we were there, the ghost identified itself as that of Kusum, a girl from Madras who had fallen in love with a young man who was subsequently compelled by his parents to marry someone else. Kusum committed suicide, and as a ghost she delighted in afflicting young men. (2010: 243–244)

This is but one of many cases from Balaji that have been recorded, and the anthropological literature is full of similar descriptions of possession in South Asia and—on this level of generalization—other parts of the world.[8] The question of how to describe, analyze, and make sense of such an example will be addressed in this article in a particular way, by discussing why it is possible for most visitors like Sanjay to experience possession shortly after arriving at Balaji. This was an observation of our research team, and similar observations have been made by Pakaslahti, who noted how patients "learn quickly" the illness and treatment discourse prevalent at Balaji with the help of the healers and more experienced patients on the basis that "most new help-seekers have some culturally shared knowledge of the concept of spirit illness and its basic expressions" (2008: 159). But what kinds of "knowledge" do they possess? Would we three researchers from Heidelberg University also have been able to become possessed after acquiring the same knowledge with the help of the healers and more experienced patients? There is no doubt that most visitors to Balaji have been familiar with possession for a long time, since childhood.[9] If so, what aspects of their socialization could count as necessary conditions to be able to "comply" with the particular responses that institutions such as Balaji call forth in order to start the therapeutic processes? How can these conditions be described and theorized?

In the following it will be argued that in order to understand how help seekers like Sanjay are able to comply so quickly with the practices of institutions like Balaji, their specific "background" has to be understood. To some degree this background can be fruitfully described by comparing and interrelating the ways in which the anthropologist McKim Marriott opposes individuals to "dividuals," and how the philosopher Charles Taylor contrasts "buffered selves" living in a secular world to "porous selves" living in an enchanted world. At the end of this chapter it will be argued, however, that Marriott's and Taylor's insights have to be unhinged from their larger theoretical frameworks, and that they can be related fruitfully to Bourdieu's notion of "habitus" and complemented with recent anthropological studies of "learning possession." On this basis the article suggests that further research should focus particularly on the ways in which many people are able to "comply" with the demands of healing temples as well as OPDs by making culturally informed choices on the basis of heterogeneous sets of cultural expertise, without ignoring that such choices can have far-reaching and problematic consequences for them (as pointed out by Naraindas, this volume).

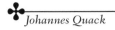

Marriott: Dividuals and Possession

In Chicago in the 1970s, anthropologist McKim Marriott developed a metatheoretical approach that he labeled "ethnosociology." Its central postulate is that any analysis of a foreign culture should only apply categories that belong to that culture, and must therefore begin by investigating "the ontology of that culture" (1992: 269). The motto of this approach is also the title of a book edited by Marriott: *India through Hindu Categories* (1990b).[10] As a first approximation one has to understand his ethnosociological approach as a challenge to the universal applicability of Western analytical terms and concepts and a plea to identify and apply "emic" terms and concepts instead. But Marriott's aims go further and can be separated into two steps, which he constructs as analogs to developments within the field of (universal) linguistics. The central problem Marriott detects is that for a long time, languages (cultures) had been explained and understood by employing the alleged universality of Latin grammar (Western social sciences). But while in linguistics the scientists realized that it is more fruitful and adequate to investigate "ethno-grammars" in their own right, this insight was not reached in the social sciences with respect to non-Western cultures. Accordingly Marriott suggests establishing a "general but alternative social science for India," i.e., an alternative to the social sciences inherited from Marx, Weber, Durkheim, and the rest of the social science pantheon. The anthropologist L. A. Babb points out that what is at stake is "an entirely new level, the indigenisation of theory itself" (1990: 203). In order to accomplish this, Marriot, influenced by the work of David Schneider, tried to trace "irreducible elements and units" of the Indian (and by extension any other) cultural system in order to apply only these analytical concepts, so that no category contradicts the ontological commitments on which the respective culture is based (see Marriott and Inden 1977: 232). He proposed to do the same for any other non-Western culture. In a second step—which Marriott never actually took—he envisioned combining all established ethnosociologies to one "truly general social science," which would not be limited to one culture (be it Europe or India) but would comprise all cultures just as a "general science of linguistics began to develop only with the writing of alternative grammars" (1992: 269).[11]

The contribution Marriott made toward the first step through his attempt to establish an ethnosociology of India encompasses three central theoretical concepts ("Indian categories"): nonduality, transactions, and dividuals, which I will briefly introduce here.[12] The first alternative concept introduced by Marriott is that of *nonduality*.[13] He argues that in the Indian context it makes no sense to differentiate in a Cartesian fashion between mind and body. This is exemplified by Marriott with the notion of *dharma,* which is often conceptualized as a moral code of conduct, religious guideline, or law. According to Marriott, *dharma* is better understood as something material as well as conceptual, as made up of "substance codes" related to an "embodied morality." His point is that in India the exchange of bodily and other substances can influence one's moral and religious qualities. The affiliation to a *jāti* (the endogamous sections of Hindu society usually translated as caste) or *kūla* (lineage) is, among other things, determined through exchange of "coded bodily substances," i.e., of something that is at the same time material as well as moral. Against dualistic theories Marriott attempted to visualize his alternative approach through a three-dimensional cube that features the axis: *mixing, marking,* and *matching* with their respective oppositions *unmixing, unmarking,* and *unmatching.* This highly complex and controversial concept became somewhat comprehensible to me in Marriott's article "The Female Family Core Explored Ethnosociologically" (1998) while Zimmerman's article (this volume) interprets and employs this triad in a fruitful and convincing way (see also Rosin 2000).

How this system of exchange of coded bodily substances works is described by Marriott under the label of *transactions.* Rejecting Dumont's all-encompassing structural opposition between (religious/ritual) purity and impurity, Marriott stresses that this opposition is only one element of a much larger transactional system that can best exemplified by analyses of the Indian caste system. The everyday practices of exchange of food, service, money, words, etc., constitute caste hierarchies rather than abstract attributions along a pure-impure scale (like "meat-eater"), which are neither consistent nor reliable when it comes to the actual specification of caste hierarchies.[14]

Since Marriott's third concept of *dividuals* as opposed to the Western idea of in-dividuals will be discussed further below, it will suffice here to quote from his own summary: "Correspondingly, persons—single actors—are not thought in South Asia to be 'individual,' that is, indivisible, bounded units, as they are in much of Western social and psychological theory as well as in common sense. Instead, it appears that persons are generally thought by South Asians to be 'dividual' or divisible. To exist, dividual persons absorb heterogeneous material influences. They must also give out from themselves particles of their own coded substances" (Marriott 1976: 111).[15]

While the specific concepts introduced by Marriott have been applied fruitfully in various ways,[16] his larger theoretical approach was subject to strong criticism. Most relevant is a short but vehement discussion that took place in the early 1990s in the journal *Contributions to Indian Sociology*.[17] The major points of criticism include Babb's argument that Marriott developed his concepts not only on the basis of Indian preferences, but also his own, given that in India there has been theorizing of many kinds ignored by Marriott who primarily focused on the influence of the Samkhya tradition (1990: 202). Most significant for me is that Marriott commits cross-culturally the same "positivistic" mistake committed by the nineteenth-century historicism of Leopold von Ranke, Friedrich Meinecke, and others. Like Marriott with respect to India, they tried to characterize the particularity of the ancient Greeks. Although they were less concerned with the governing ontological assumptions of Greek culture, they share Marriott's positivistic ideal of descriptions that are not influenced and prejudiced by one's own (contemporary and "Western") position; they sought instead to "understand Homer through Homerian categories" (Landfester 2002: 98, my translation), an attempt that was thoroughly criticized in the nineteenth-century by Friedrich Nietzsche and later expanded by the philosopher Hans-Georg Gadamer. What Gadamer argues for in terms of historical understanding holds equally true for cross-cultural approaches. Gadamer outlines in great sophistication that "prejudices" or "pre-judgments" (*Vorurteile*) are a necessary condition for any kind of understanding and that history (read Marriott's "culture") is not merely an object of inquiry like any object of the natural sciences. History does not belong to us, but we belong to history. Truly, historical thinking must reflect its own history. It is only if we stop chasing the phantom of a historical object that can be described independent of our own position that we will learn to recognize in the object that which differentiates the other from the self and thereby understand the other as well as the self (see Gadamer 1990: 281, 305).

The attempt to establish a "general social science" for all cultures has been questioned more and more in the last few decades and was considered "anachronistic" even by Marriott's students (Daniel 1984: 54). Having said this, it is worth noting that other aspects of Marriott's approach antedated related approaches in the social sciences. His statement that the "imperial style of Western ethnosocial science excludes competing definitions of reality from its published reports" (1990a: 4), for example, is not altogether different from the much later attempt of scholars such as Dipesh Chakrabarty to establish "subaltern histories" (2000). As noted already by Marriott's student E. Valentine Daniel, the most important insight of Marriott's ethnosociology might be that "[r]egardless of how much we may ethnocize anthropological theory, anthropology will be part of the Western or Westernized intellectual's symbolic system" (1984: 54). Indeed, Daniel's definition of ethnosociology as operating "paradoxically: as hoping to reach a goal it hopes never to reach" is not altogether different from Chakrabarty's observations that in his and the larger postcolonial approach "European thought is at once both indispensable and inadequate" (2000: 16) and the "everyday paradox" of the non-Western scholar that "*we* find these theories, in spite of their inherent ignorance of 'us,' eminently useful in understanding our societies" (2000: 29).

Reflecting on these issues and debates I suggest that we should value and apply the ethnographic insights of Marriott as well as his argument that contemporary everyday life in India can be better understood if Indian philosophical and cosmological concepts are taken into account, without buying into his more problematic metatheoretical attempts. Some of the points raised by Gerow (2000), the contribution of Zimmermann to this volume as well as the wider application of his key concepts within anthropology are evidence enough of the productivity of Marriott's insights. In this respect, the his concept of dividuals came to be accepted widely in scholarly work on South Asia, not the least in interpretations of possession-practices. In his engrossing volume *The Self Possessed* the Sanskritist Frederick Smith argues, for example, that "although Marriott has applied this concept to caste transactions, the question 'How does possession work?' can be answered in part through application of his concept" (2006: 75). Reference to Marriott and his students Daniel and Lamb with respect to possession can also be found in Fabrega's *History of Mental Illness in India* (2009: 610–611). Yet, neither of them elaborates further on the specific ways in which the insights of Marriott are instrumental in attempts to explain the phenomenon of possession. This is what I propose to do in what follows.

The anthropologist Grace Gredys Harris notes that Marriott's writing implies that for Indian dividuals, the content of their bio-social bodies varies greatly given that elements of the Hindu world flow in and out of a human being so as to make the latter an almost constantly changing configuration. But she also assesses that Marriott thereby conflates the categories of individual and person (1989: 601). In that respect she suggests using the concept of the *individual* as referring to a human being considered as a single member of the humankind, with the body marking the physical boundaries of individuals (and death its biological end). To be a *person* in the full sense of the term, as suggested by Harris, can be described by drawing on what Max Weber called "subjective meaning" (*subjektiver Sinn*), i.e., the central characteristic of an intentional action (and opposed to mere behavior).[18] However, this criticism does injustice to Marriott's position since the fusion of biology and sociomoral aspects necessarily follows from his observation that in India, actions are not only "social" but always imply something "substantial" and "biological" because they generally change the actor's substance-code. *Dharma* does not only denote "law" or "order," but is as much a biophysical category as it is a sociomoral one. The "coded-substances" of an individual (biological) are crucially defined by actions as persons (social).

If one applies the crucial insights of Marriott to analyses of possession, then what is usually called the possessing "spirit" must not be understood as merely some metaphysical or psychological entity. Like the notion of *dharma*, the notions central to understandings of possession, most famously that of *bhūt* but also *ātma* ("self") or *havā* ("wind"), have to be understood as simultaneously substantial, psychological, moral, spiritual, and social.[19] Shifting from concepts to practices it becomes all the more obvious that the most common ways in which one becomes afflicted, as well as the modes in which affliction is manifested, experienced, and therapeutically dealt with, depend on the exchange of coded substances. The two

main and non-mutually-exclusive modes of affliction as differentiated by Pakaslahti on the basis of his data from Balaji are found
all over North India and can be taken hereby as exemplary of this
point. Possession is generally explained either as being in the wrong
place at the wrong time or as intentionally caused by someone. The
latter, intentionally caused, affliction is often seen as brought about
by "ensorcelled" food or drink or by stepping upon "cursed" items,
for example a lemon sprinkled with vermillion and turmeric, inside
a piece of cloth folded from the four corners inward, that might
have been "read upon" (i.e., powerful formulas being uttered during
preparation). Impersonal sources of affliction are especially associated with liminal places like thresholds and crossroads, and liminal
times when the body is generally "open" and vulnerable to unwanted
exchanges of substances, for example when urinating, during and
after sex, at the time of menstruation or during the period following
a family member's death, as well as with impure places like ceme-
teries and cremation grounds. Such ideas and experiences are widespread and embedded in the everyday lives of many Indians.

Marriott's description of the ways in which the borders that define
human beings can be more or less transactional or fluid does not
mean that dividuals do not have a sense of themselves as separate
beings, as Obeyesekere puts it (1990: 249). In the example given
above, the "victim" of spirit possession (Sanjay) and the intruding
"spirit" (Kusum) are two distinct entities. A striking illustration of
this point can be found in Sax's report of how a deceased mother
possesses her daughter Devaki and speaks through her body to the
guru and the other family members present. "After some time the
mother's ghost asks after her daughter Devaki, and one of the other
women there informs her that it is actually Devaki whom she has
possessed, and through whom she has been speaking" (2009: 194).
For the people present it is obvious that both cannot be present at
the same time. Further, neither Devaki nor Sanjay is later taken to
be responsible for what was said and done by the possessing spirit
through his or her body.[20] In fact, in general it is especially important
for the ritual healer to find out who is currently speaking and acting,
what the spirits' reasons for possession are, and whether these can
be met through offerings or vows. The crucial relevance of Marriott's
focus on biomoral transactions between dividuals with respect to this
article is to see that the experiences as well as the interpretations of

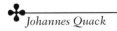
possession in India are based on the exchange of coded substances. In the following we will see the way in which Charles Taylor's differentiation between "porous" and "buffered selves" contributes to this issue.

Taylor: Porous Selves and Possession

Charles Taylor, the author of an impressive list of books including the classic *Sources of the Self: The Making of Modern Identity* (1992), capped his long academic career as a philosopher with the publication of his voluminous and distinguished *A Secular Age* (2007). In this opus magnum he attempts to describe the "background" of a secular age as "the whole context of understanding in which our moral, spiritual or religious experience and search takes place" (2007: 3). A secular age is thereby opposed by Taylor to an enchanted world in which spirits, moral forces, things, and words can transform independently of human beings, and where the line between personal agency and impersonal force, as well as between the physical and the moral, is not impermeable. In a way that is remarkably similar to Marriott, Taylor argues that experiences of certain boundaries in an enchanted world—for example between "humans and things" and between "mind and world"—are experienced as porous and he therefore speaks of those living in this world as having "porous selves." This "porousness is most clearly in evidence in the fear of possession," which has to be seen, however, primarily as a fact of *experience,* not only as a matter of theory or belief (2007: 35). With respect to the issue of possession Taylor goes as far as to note that "we tend to think of our differences from our remote forbears in terms of different beliefs, whereas there is something much more puzzling involved here. It is clear that for our forbears, and many people in the world today who live in a similar religious world, the presence of spirits, and of different forms of possession, is no more a matter of (optional, voluntarily embraced) belief than is for me the presence of this computer and its keyboard at the tips of my fingers" (Taylor 2008, accessed 3 March 2012: para. 6). In opposition to Marriott, Taylor makes very explicit here that we are not just dealing with different conceptualizations.[21] Living in an enchanted world as opposed to a disenchanted one is for Taylor primarily a difference in the ways in which people experience the world. In his many publications Taylor speaks of "background understanding," "background sense," and "background practices."[22] Here I will follow his use of the term in *A Secular Age* where he draws on ideas developed by illustrious scholars such as Heidegger, Merleau-Ponty, Wittgenstein, Michael Polanyi, as well as John Searle and Hubert Dreyfus (both of whom also use the term "background")[23] in order to argue for certain conditions for the possibility of making sense of the world by ordering everyday reality (see 2007: 14, 172–174, 323–325). The basic argument is that explicit thoughts and everyday practices can only be entertained or performed against an unformulated (and perhaps in part unformulable) background sense of who and where we are in the world and among other beings. For Taylor, the crucial reference points for any human "background" are the world, others, time, and the moral realm. "This relation can, indeed, be transformed as we move from one culture or age to another, but it cannot just fall away. We cannot be without some sense of our moral situation, some sense of our connectedness to others" (1995: 32). For the buffered self, it is crucial for its way of being in the world that these boundaries are experienced as closed. In fact, this closedness on the background level, according to Taylor, is the necessary condition for the development of theories of the mind as separate from the body. Be that as it may, Taylor and Marriott present us with two bipolar types of the self; taken together the buffered individual can be contrasted with the porous dividual. While this opposition is very illustrative, its shortcomings will be discussed in the reminder of this chapter.

Against Bipolar Types

Out of the widespread discussions of the concepts of individual, person, and self in anthropological literature, probably the most oft-quoted statement was made by Clifford Geertz, who characterized the Western concept of the self as "peculiar" in that it is "a bounded, unique, more or less integrated motivational and cognitive universe, a dynamic centre of awareness, emotion, judgment, and action organized into a distinctive whole and set contrastively against other such wholes and against its social and natural background" (Geertz 1983: 59). Geertz is not the only one to make such a point. Above it was argued that Marriott and Taylor argue roughly along similar lines given their opposition between the buffered individual of the secular West and the porous dividuals of the enchanted "Rest."[24]

Yet, it would be as treacherous to ignore the different religious settings within the Western world, where various kinds of possession experiences are common, as it would be naive to assume that possession experiences are naturally occurring and taken-for-granted phenomena for all Indians. There are many people in India for whom possession is a rather "exotic" phenomenon and there are people who explicitly argue that all such instances are either an expression of a mental disorder, or an example of dissimulation. Concerning the latter group, I conducted an ethnographic study on one specific organization called *Andhashraddha Nirmulan Samiti* (Society for the Eradication of Superstition, ANiS) in Maharashtra (Quack 2012b). A central aspect of my fieldwork consisted of traveling with ANiS activists and their "science vans" to villages, schools, and colleges where they staged programs with the aim of spreading a scientific worldview and "scientific temper"[25] in order to constrain and eradicate "superstitious" beliefs and practices. One part of the program always featured the performance of "magic tricks" on the basis of which some religious specialists in India—whom the rationalists refer to as "godmen"—are credited with supernatural powers. The rationalists expose the tricks by giving explanations of how they are performed. The central message is that there are no miracles and supernatural forces in the world, that in principle everything can be explained by science. A second part of the program attempts to explain why many Indians believe in spirits that are able to possess humans. In order to do so they refer to theories of how the human mind functions and outline their perspectives on the connection between mental health issues and beliefs in spirit possession. During these programs they outline why they consider people who show signs of possession either as mentally ill or dissimulating.

Since the criticism of possession rituals was so central to the aims and activities of the rationalists, I had many discussions with ANiS activists on this topic. It was obvious that the idea of becoming possessed was rather alien to them. In general there was no reason to describe them either as dividuals or as porous. They did not assume that spirits, moral forces, things, and words can transform the world independently of human beings. Ancestors, spirits, and other such entities did not play any role in their social world. For them the world is constituted by material elements, standing in a cause-and-effect relationship, and hence they argue that the world is—in principle—explainable, and therefore controllable (to paraphrase Weber's famous description of "disenchantment"). They were lacking any "sense" for possession experiences in the cognitive as well as physical meaning of the word (see Quack 2010: 182).

In the Western world—to follow the opposition set up explicitly by Geertz and more implicitly by Marriott and Taylor—descriptions of contemporary possession experiences are to be found in eclectic sources such as popular films (e.g., *The Exorcist*), specific psychiatric studies (e.g., Pfeifer 1994), or detailed ethnographies (e.g., Csordas 1997; for a comparative overview, see Csordas and Lewton 1998). To be mentioned here in particular is a study by Tanja Luhrmann on witches in contemporary Great Britain (1989) because it can be seen as a positive/negative counterpoint to the study of the Indian rationalists (Quack 2012b) given that stereotypical representations of a disenchanted Europe and an enchanted India ignore the existence of their respective counterexamples. Spiro makes a relevant point here: the "bipolar types of self—a Western and a non-Western—are wildly overdrawn" and "there is much more differentiation, individuation, and autonomy in the putative non-Western self, and much more dependence and interdependence in the putative Western self, than these binary opposite types allow" (1993: 117). Harris rightly adds that "in societies that are internally differentiated socially and culturally . . . there are differing, competing conceptualizations of individual, self, and person" (1989: 608; for a similar point, see Ewing 1990).

At the same time it can hardly be ignored that possession is much more common in India compared to contemporary Western countries where reports of such experiences seem to have steadily declined in a larger historical perspective. The challenge is to theorize these differences without generalizing too much about bipolar types of self, i.e., by refining the picture painted by Marriott and Taylor with the rather broad strokes of their conceptual brushes. In the remainder of the chapter, exemplary approaches are discussed to explore the ways in which it may be helpful to complement the argument about "porous dividuals" with finer conceptual tools. This is done by differentiating between two levels: the first level relates back to Taylor's notion of the "background." His argumentation will

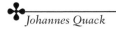

be complemented with the work on types of religiosities and subjectivities by Saba Mahmood. On the second level the focus will be
on personal experiences and processes of learning as researched in
cognitive anthropology in particular.

For the sake of completeness it can be added that many ethnographies stress multisensorial performances and special settings that
facilitate particular possession experiences. Indeed, while Mehen-
dipur is by and large an average Indian city, the atmosphere around
Balaji healing temple and at the *samādhi-sthal* is notably different.
First of all, people either come with great expectation or, after successful healing experiences, leave with great gratitude. At any given
time of day we visited the *samādhi-sthal,* dozens of people ritually
circled the tomb, many of whom were dissociated, besotted, ver-
tiginous, possessed, in trance, or just "spaced-out." We saw smaller
groups of people in intense conversation about ongoing healing
practices; larger groups of people would sing and clap their hands
in encouragement while accompanying and dealing with spirits and
gods taking possession of family members or friends. Inside Balaji
healing temple the experience is even more intense: "The senses are
taken hold of violently and wrenched out of their normal grooves
by strange sights and unfamiliar sounds and smells, embedded in
a whirling crowd of pilgrims, patients and their families in various
stages of self-absorption" (Kakar 1982: 60). These are the words of
the psychoanalyst Sudhir Kakar, who also noted "the wide gulf in the
range of behavior permitted and encouraged [at Balaji] as compared
to rooms and spaces where every-day life is carried on" and which
is "very different from the solemnity of a modern psychotherapist's
office" (1982: 63). But while such distinct atmospheres and settings
may be conducive to possession experiences, the question remains
as to why the respective triggers do not work equally well for all
people, why people like Sanjay are able to comply so easily to the
practices Balaji asks for.

Background, Subjectivities, Learning, and Habitus

How are possession experiences linked to epistemological and ontological assumptions that are embodied in people's everyday lives
and institutionalized in normative conceptions of subjectivities and

semiotics? Questions at such a fundamental level were raised by Taylor and answered with reference to the concept of "background." This line of inquiry can be further refined by looking at some recent anthropological writing, for example, those who work in the tradition of Talal Asad. In his writing on the mutually constitutive nature of "the secular" and "the religious" Asad (following Wittgenstein) outlines how these concepts and the related practices can be indicative of different background "grammars" that constitute different landscapes of power (moral, political, economic) and enable or foreclose specific behaviors, knowledges, and sensibilities (Asad 2003: 25, 36, 48). Following Asad's approach, Saba Mahmood, for example, tries to trace the ways in which religious and secular worldviews are related to each other by looking—in broad agreement with Taylor—not only at "beliefs," but at normative conceptions of the subject and language as well as related cultivations of bodily attitudes, virtues, habits, and desires within the practices of everyday life (see Mahmood 2005, especially 45–48). Mahmood contrasts two kinds of subjectivity that emerged from different "backgrounds" or "grammars," specified by her by different embodied understandings, e.g., of exteriority, interiority, autonomy, and agency as well as semiotics. Her argument concerning the latter was antedated by scholars like J. P. S. Uberoi (whose work is not mentioned by Mahmood); both consider the reformed reinterpretation of religious objects (such as the host) as a paradigmatic instance. Here it becomes most obvious how religious objects came to be seen as standing in for the divine through an act of human encoding and interpretation (as mere "symbols" or "signs"), as opposed to "embodiments of the divine," e.g., as the "real presence" (*Realpräsenz*) of Jesus Christ in flesh and blood (see Uberoi 1978: 28–32). In contrast to the protestant-secular position, Mahmood argues that "natives" attributed "divine agency to material signs, often regarded material objects (and their exchange) as an ontological extension of themselves (thereby dissolving the distinction between persons and things)" (2009: 844). Implicitly evoking some of the central points of Taylor and Marriott outlined above, Mahmood argues that such subjectivities do not categorically differentiate in a Cartesian fashion between mind and body, or between humans and things, material and moral, signifier and signified. Their respective religiosity is not based on a set of propositions that one has personal reasons to believe or not. Rather, the particular

71

(enchanted) "mode of religiosity"[26] Mahmood describes consists of embodied morality and piety cultivated through rituals and liturgy, and is based on codes of conduct, and—in the Islamic case—on the culture of the *ummah* and submission to Allah. As in Taylor's case, Mahmood tries to ascribe to the prereflective background, a certain way of understanding the world, oneself, and one's social relationships to other beings in this world.

Given that Mahmood's contrast between a secularized mode of religiosity as opposed to an "unenlightened form of religiosity" (2005: xiv) has considerable overlaps with the binary set up by Taylor, it is important to note that Mahmood questions her own binary theorizing.[27] She notes that the kind of religiosity she is looking at is not representative of a specific time (premodern) or space (non-modern) but has gained its specific shape by processes of secularization and various pushes to reform within Egypt's cultural history and transcultural exchanges (2005: 44–45).[28] In contrast to Taylor and especially Marriott, Mahmood explicitly rejects the assumption of "a homogeneous notion of a self that is coextensive with a given culture or temporality." Rather she tries to show how "very different configurations of personhood can cohabit the same cultural and historical space" (2005: 120). Finally, Mahmood also challenges a binary that is addressed in this volume at large, that between the logic of subversion and/or consolidation of (therapeutic) asymmetries and their underlying normative orders. In critical engagement with the work of Bourdieu, she argues that a simple focus on subversion versus consolidation may elide "the different modalities through which the body comes to inhabit or live the regulative power of norms, modalities that cannot be captured within the dualistic logic of resistance and constraint" (2005: 27).

Mahmood further criticizes that a Bourdieuian approach lacks attention to the pedagogical process by which a "habitus" is learned not only through socialization within a specific "background" but also through conscious training (2005: 138–139). Here (and with respect to some related points)[29] I cannot agree with her. As will be shown below, it is precisely through Bourdieu's focus on habitus formation in everyday life that the two levels of analysis distinguished here can be brought together. Yet, before we turn to this argument it can be recapitulated that Mahmood's attempt is not to link her distinction among different kinds of religiosity to certain "cultures" or a certain "age," but to various normative conceptions of subjectivity and language, and the epistemological and ontological assumptions that undergird these norms. She quotes Foucault on the question of different subjectivities: "You do not have the same type of relationship to yourself when you constitute yourself as a political subject who goes to vote or speaks at a meeting and when you are seeking to fulfill your desires in a sexual relationship. Undoubtedly there are relationships and interferences between these different forms of the subject; but we are not dealing with the same type of subjects" (Foucault 1987, cited in Mahmood 2005: 121). A more Foucauldian and Asadian approach leads to an exploration of the different subjectivities that people exhibit when they visit Balaji or an OPD, and the different normative orders people (must) "comply" with in their everyday lives. In this respect it is important to note the observation made by Naraindas in this volume that moving among competing nosologies, and their associated epistemologies, may not be unproblematic for some people. His chapter illustrates that we are not dealing with an easygoing, "live-and-let-live" form of medical pluralism where people easily choose among alternative forms of therapy. Instead, every decision implies a position with respect to competing ontologies and epistemologies, be it through compliance or contestation, which may have far-reaching experiential consequences.[30]

At the second level of analysis, a theoretically diverse set of ethnographic studies all draw on the work of Bourdieu to show that people from various backgrounds can or may have to learn or acquire, as well as unlearn or lose, the knowledge and cultural dispositions necessary for possession experiences. Sax describes, for example, a family settled in Delhi who returned to their ancestral village in the mountains of Garhwal for a major healing ritual. While the father refused to attend the key events, the children were unable to participate in it properly when their turns came and, eventually, "their grandmother saved the day—and the ritual—by vigorously dancing [i.e., becoming possessed] for more than a quarter of an hour" (2009: 233). From the main argument of Sax's book it becomes clear that being able to become possessed presupposes certain "dispositions" that have been lost in this example by the younger members of the family. Sax stresses the notions of "embodiment" and argues that in possession myth and iconography, context and social memory, power and morality, all come together. He draws on his long research experience as well as Bourdieu when he further lists groups of people whose "habitus" had changed because they were no longer integrated into their traditional society: "educated professionals, emigrants to the city, military officers, NRIs (non-resident Indians) living overseas, students studying in urban universities, and the like" (2009: 49). When confronted with the possession-rituals of the hills, most of them were not able to be possessed. Sax explains this with the aid of Bourdieu's notion of the "hysteresis effect," i.e., when the practices associated with the old habitus "incur negative sanctions when the environment with which they are actually confronted is too distant from that to which they are objectively fitted . . . caus[ing] one group to experience as natural or reasonable practices or aspirations which another group finds unthinkable or scandalous, and vice versa" (Bourdieu 1977: 78). In other words, for those who have not embodied the respective myth, memory, and morality, becoming possessed is difficult or even impossible. Along similar lines, anthropologist Simpson argued how knowledge and skills connected to possession rituals that had been passed on from generation to generation by specialists within the *Bervā* caste in Sri Lanka gradually diminished because of the "classic rupture between customary, embodied modes of practice on the one hand and the drive towards modernity on the other" (1997: 44).

Yet, while some people apparently lose their ability to become possessed, others are able to consciously learn the required "knowledge." This is convincingly shown by Halloy and Naumescu's cognitive approach toward processes of "learning possession," described in terms of a *cultural expertise*, which every possessed person must gain and master if she wants her state to be socially recognized. By "expertise" they mean "first of all the culturally relevant matching or assemblage of emotion, perception and reasoning in the process of learning a determined skill. Possession for example, requires an expertise both from the observers, who perceive it in relation to shared social values and aesthetic and normative criteria offered by that particular culture, and from the possessed person who has to make sense of her own experience" (2012: 166).

Halloy and Naumescu describe the learning of possession as an open-ended process that is not just about "matching" cultural expectations with bodily states and perceptual skills, but also learning to "play up" with them. In line with what is argued here they analyze the necessary "fine-tuning of attention, perception and action" as giving birth to what Bourdieu called *body hexis,* i.e., the bodily memory and motoric schemes according to which our bodies are conditioned to act (2012: 168).[31]

In order to bring the two levels of background and learning together one may speak of a dispositional cultural expertise that is not only learned in specific learning environments, but also acquired through socialization in institutionalized normative orders with distinct epistemologies and ontologies. The respective experiences and interpretations of possession are reinforced by, and reinforce themselves through, institutions where possession is "asked for," such as Balaji. The co-constitutive nature of experiences, ideas, and institutions is able to establish and to perpetuate a more or less consistent system of ideas and practices about the world and human beings' place in it. By combining the insights of Marriott and Taylor we can formulate the argument that the notion of "porous dividuals" describes one particularly favorable background for the possibility of experiencing possession. The respective ability to experience possession is not primarily based on certain beliefs but is constituted through experiences of constant sociomoral and religious exchanges of coded substances that enter and leave the body. The way one is afflicted by, and gets rid of, "spirits" in places like Balaji is consistent with, as well as reinforced by, various aspects of the everyday lives of most visitors. Sanjay's experience of possession is to be seen in Taylor's approach as a specific existential condition, shaped through bodily dispositions and the ideas, practices, and institutions with which he grew up.

Yet, there is no reason to assume that any given background is necessarily homogenous and clear-cut, that people grow up within only one set of institutionalized normative orders and its respective ideas and practices, i.e., that people establish only one kind of cultural expertise. The triad of ideas, practices, and institutions is not as static and clear-cut as Marriott's and Taylor's approaches suggest; boundaries between therapies are contested, circumvented, and blurred in many ways. One must look at not only the situations in which possession occurs or does not occur, but at the processes of explicit or diffuse learning that are taking place within everyday life, where people in contemporary India as well as elsewhere are often exposed to very heterogeneous milieus. What is often called "medical pluralism" in particular and the diversity of lifestyles and influences in contemporary India in general means that there are many ideas, practices, and institutions addressing issues of health and illness coexisting, competing, affecting, and transforming each other at the same time along the asymmetries outlined in this volume. What fits for one person might not fit for another (Halliburton 2004). The modes of thought and codes of conduct of the Indian rationalists with respect to health and illness do not fit to formal institutions such as the Balaji healing shrine. Yet, the rationalists are a very particular example because of their categorical stance on matters of religion. For the majority of people in contemporary India this is not a question of either-or: they might visit Balaji as well as OPD at the same time. By doing so they may get caught, however, in the imperatives, contingencies, and dilemmas resulting from their respective therapeutic choices (see Naraindas, this volume).

How many patients become possessed by a spirit, deceased relative, god, or goddess in the OPD of a psychiatric clinic in India? Very few, if any. Many Indians establish the capacity to exhibit the appropriate codes of conduct in different therapeutic institutions such as a healing temple or a psychiatric ward (leaving aside the various religious and medical settings where such codes are blurred in the first place). On the basis of their heterogeneous background they may acquire the bodily and cognitive knowledge and dispositions that enable them to "play both games," so as to comply in some degree with the practical demands of Balaji and OPD.[32] Yet, they might not freely choose between these different therapeutic offers, and there is the danger of getting lost in translation between competing therapeutic constructions of the world based on different "metaphysical premises" (Naraindas, this volume) or "grammars" (Asad), given that these grammars have the potential to open up or close very different possibilities for acting and being (Asad 2003: 73). Further, they might not have the same type of relationship to their "self" when they constitute themselves as biomedical patients in the OPD and when they are possessed by a god, goddess, or spirit. Yet, this does not mean that there are no relationships or interferences between these different forms of the subject. The institutions, ideas, and practices that constitute the kinds of persons people take and experience themselves to be are not necessarily representative of one master-category. Many people in India (or elsewhere) cannot be described either as secular subjects of biopower or as religious subjects of other traditions, as buffered individuals or as porous dividuals; by exhibiting different and blurred subjectivities and by bearing the resulting experiential opportunities and predicaments they try to deal with the demands of both Balaji and OPD.

Acknowledgments

The research was conducted from February to November 2010 as part of the research project "Asymmetrical Translations: Mind and Body in European and Indian Medicine" at the University of Heidelberg. It was financed by the Cluster of Excellence, "Asia and Europe in a Global Context" (Excellence Initiative of the German Research Foundation). I would like to thank the three anonymous reviewers as well as Eva Jansen, Claudia Lang, Harish Naraindas, and William S. Sax for very helpful comments on previous versions of this chapter and Ahmed Nabil for proofreading the English.

Notes

1. The group of people who had difficulties conforming to all these demands will be the subject of a different publication.
2. For the social background of the visitors see Dwyer (2003: 159), discussed and supplemented by Pakaslahti (2005).
3. As with many similar places in India and elsewhere, the help and therapy offered at Balaji healing temple is not restricted to "psychology": all sorts of problems can be dealt with, be they physical, psychological, social, spiritual, or all of the above. Yet Satija et al. (1982) argued that 92 percent of the help seekers in Balaji suffered from diagnosable psychiatric illnesses, assessed mostly as neurotic disorders (quoted in Pakaslahti 2009: 156).
4. See Kakar (1982), Dwyer (2003), Pakaslahti (1998, 2005, 2009), and Sax and Weinhold (2010).
5. For a description of the "divine landscape" at Balaji, see, e.g., Kakar (1982: 57–60) and Pakaslahti (1998: 135–138).
6. The practices and psychosocial and professional characteristics of healers coming and staying at Balaji in addition to those of the local priests are well described by Pakaslahti (2005: 220–224).
7. *Āratī* is an honorific passing of a flame (lighted lamp, piece of camphor, etc.) in a circular, clockwise fashion in front of a deity.
8. For a general overview, see Boddy (1994), and for a detailed overview of South Asia, see Smith (2006).
9. On the one hand it is striking to see how quickly people "learn possession" at places like Balaji. My visits to similar healing places in Maharashtra, Gujarat, Rajasthan, and Uttarakhand, on the other hand, showed me that

the bodily movements and signs that often accompany possession experiences can be quite similar across India.

10. The applications of Marriott's ethnosociology to Japan and Morocco (see 1992) remained very preliminary.

11. Such an idea can be traced back to the influence Edwards Shils and Talcott Parsons had on him. Marriott seeks to "do for India what they did for Europe" following the Parsons and Shils method all the way to constructing "an alternative general theoretical system for the social sciences of a non-Western civilization" (1990a: 5). As Parsons developed a sociological theory as a synthesis of the several classical analytical concepts derived from Western sociologists in the Chicago of the 1960s and '70s, Marriott aims at expanding this attempt to the whole world.

12. A further concept stressed by Marriott and his followers is that of "fluidity," which is deeply interconnected to that of dividuals. One of Marriott's students, the anthropologist Sarah Lamb, focuses particularly on the fluidity of gender oppositions. She shows with great ethnographic sensitivity how women can get "cooler" and "more closed" in the process of aging and thereby more and more like men. She writes that "persons have more or less open boundaries and may therefore affect one another's natures through transaction of food, services, words, bodily substances, and the like" (2000: 31).

13. Below I engage with some criticisms of Marriott's position. Here I only want to mention that Wendy Doniger (O'Flaherty) refers of all people to A. K. Ramanujan—who contributed to Marriott's volume *India through Hindu Categories* (1990)—on the point that "dualism is an (if not the) Indian way of thinking" (2009: 11). Given that Marriott, Doniger, and Ramanujan taught together at the University of Chicago, this can only be understood as an implicit but conscious rebuttal of Marriott's claim that nonduality is one central characteristic of India.

14. In line with what has been said above on nonduality, Lamb elaborately describes how the concept of *maya*, understood as a "web of attachments, affections, jealousies, and love that in Bengalis' eyes make up social relations," is made up of "codes of conduct" and "transactions" that establish *maya* as a "net of bodily-emotional ties" (2000: 28).

15. In the much-celebrated book *The Gender of the Gift* Marilyn Strathern introduces the notion of "dividuals" as well, albeit without reference to Marriott and with a somewhat different focus. Strathern contrasts Western ideas of the "individual" (as opposed to "society") to Melanesian dividuals, who "contain a generalized sociality within" (1988: 13). Saba Mahmood notes that she shares Strathern's aim of displacing "Western analytical categories by staging inversions of familiar ways of thinking and conceptualizing" (Mahmood 2005: 190). This focus, as will be outlined below when discussing the work of Mahmood, indicates further differences from Marriott's approach.

16. For a detailed discussion of "transactionality," see Daniel (1984: 70–71, 124–128, 134–135); about how people perceive the recycling processes of

waste disposal see Rosin (2000); concerning the logics of the Hindu food hierarchy see Osella and Osella (2008) and Moreno and Marriott (1990); as well as Moore (1990) for further applications of Marriott's approach.

17. See the contributions by Babb (1990), Moffatt (1990), Östör and Fruzzetti (1991), and Marriott (1991).

18. In addition to offering this conceptualization of the individual and person, Harris argues that the notion of a specific *self* is demarcated by psychology rather than biology. Here the attention shifts from the physical boundaries to the locus of human experience, which centrally includes the "experience of that human's own someoneness" (1989: 601). It is important for Harris to outline that concepts of individual, self, and person attend to distinct yet related matters. She shows how this should be understood with reference to Goffman's description of "total institutions." Goffman describes how in "concentration camps, maximum security prisons, restricted wards in mental hospitals, and the like, prisoners, inmates, or patients may undergo daily and progressive public disconfirmation as agents . . ." (see 1989: 606) with possible transformations of the ways in which they experience and others conceptualize their selves. Further, she emphasizes that there are important cultural differences in the ways in which these concepts are understood and applied (1989: 607).

19. I cannot dwell at length here on the social aspects of possession and healing. This point is, however, encapsulated in Opler's often quoted insight that "Ghosts do not wander aimlessly through Indian village culture: they gather at points of stress and attack the soft spots of the social order. To follow their movements is to learn a good deal about the social order" (1958: 566). This is also outlined in great ethnographic detail by Sax (2009).

20. Interestingly, it is—to my knowledge—never discussed why people do not perform "cleaning rituals" or something similar after all the "polluting" actions that have been performed by an afflicting spirit. It is probably because the body is also not the person's body, but the spirit's body and the pollution therefore is removed when the spirit leaves.

21. For a discussion of Marriott's account of a "cultural representation" of the self see Ewing (1990: 256).

22. The problem with this terminological inconsistency is particularly far-reaching with the term practice. The question is whether any given background is the precondition for theoretical and practical activity or whether practice is what happens at the background level and therefore is the precondition of thought and action.

23. For a good comparison of the difference between Dreyfus's understanding of "background" as opposed to that of Searl, see Wrathall (2000).

24. A more extensive criticism of this opposition has been provided elsewhere with respect to the work of Taylor (Quack 2012b: 36–39).

25. The notion "scientific temper" was famously introduced to Indian public discourse by Jawaharlal Nehru. Under the government of his daughter Indira Gandhi (during the period of emergency rule) the Indian Constitution was amended with article 51-A entitled "Fundamental duties" which,

in section 51-A(h), states that all Indian citizens have a duty "to develop the scientific temper, humanism and the spirit of inquiry and reform" as per the Forty-second Amendment Act, 1976.

26. Mahmood speaks of a "kind of religiosity" (Mahmood 2005: 75, 2009: 852) whereas it might be more fruitful to differentiate between modes of religiosity (Quack 2013) and various modes of nonreligiosity or unbelief (Quack 2012b: 19–28, 271–284; 2012a) by drawing on the work of Berner (2004), not on Whitehouse (2004).

27. Mahmood also argues that her juxtaposition of the practices of the pietists against secular-liberal understandings of agency, body, and authority was not chosen by but thrust upon her. This is the perspective which, according to her, "will inevitably structure my audience's reading of this book" (Mahmood 2005: 191) and therefore this perspective has to be addressed, if only to displace its underlying assumptions.

28. In contrast to Taylor, who focuses on the growing concern with Reform (with a capital R, capturing the general decrease in the gap between the religiosity of the elites and laypeople, not just explicit reform movements) that is peculiar to Latin Christendom (Taylor 2007: 61–88).

29. Mahmood tries to challenge the fundamentals of classical action-theory, which she describes as an "Enlightenment model in which desires (sometimes along with volition) were considered to be the necessary antecedents of action" (2005: 126n. 110). Against this perspective she argues that in her model, desire "is not the *antecedent* to, or cause of, moral action, but its *product*" (2005: 126). But the fact that actions may at times produce desires does not rule out that these are caused by desires at the same time. In fact, Mahmood's descriptions of actions in her book are good examples of how specific desires (e.g., to realize God's will) cause people to take certain actions.

30. Material and experiential consequences of the underlying asymmetries have also been noted by Asad, not with respect to the idea of apparently easy and free (health care) choices but with respect to the idea of "free speech" in the public sphere (2003: 183–184).

31. These observations can be further complemented with other studies of "learning" in the anthropological literature (for a summary see Luhrmann, Nusbaum et al. 2010: 67).

32. This is akin to the "conceptual bilingualism" (Naraindas 2006: 2659), exhibited by Ayurvedic doctors in contemporary India, who having been trained in both allopathy and Ayurveda are seemingly able to straddle both systems.

References

Asad, Talal. 2003. *Formations of the Secular: Christianity, Islam, Modernity.* Stanford: Stanford University Press.

Babb, Lawrence A. 1990. "Social Science Inside Out." *Contributions to Indian Sociology* 24(2): 201–213.

Berner, Ulrich. 2004. "Modes of Religiosity and Types of Conversion in Medieval Europe and Modern Africa." In *Theorizing Religions Past: Archeology, History and Cognition,* ed. Harvey Whitehouse and Luther H. Martin. Walnut Creek, C.A.: AltaMira Press, 157–172.

Boddy, Janice. 1994. "Spirit Possession Revisited: Beyond Instrumentality." *Annual Review of Anthropology* 23(1): 407–434.

Bourdieu, Pierre. 1977. *Outline of a Theory of Practice.* Cambridge, U.K.: Cambridge University Press.

Chakrabarty, Dipesh. 2000. *Provincializing Europe: Postcolonial Thought and Historical Difference.* Princeton: Princeton University Press.

Csordas, Thomas J. 1997. *The Sacred Self: A Cultural Phenomenology of Charismatic Healing.* Berkeley: University of California Press.

Csordas, Thomas J., and Elizabeth Lewton. 1998. "Practice, Performance, and Experience in Ritual Healing." *Transcultural Psychiatry* 35(4): 435–512.

Daniel, E. Valentine. 1984. *Fluid Signs: Being a Person the Tamil Way.* Berkeley: University of California Press.

Doniger, Wendy. 2009. *The Hindus: An Alternative History.* London: Penguin Press.

Dwyer, Graham. 2003. *The Divine and the Demonic: Supernatural Affliction and its Treatment in North India.* London: Routledge Curzon.

Ewing, Katherine P. 1990. "The Illusion of Wholeness: Culture, Self, and the Experience of Inconsistency." *Ethos* 18(3): 251–278.

Fabrega Jr., Horacio. 2009. *History of Mental Illness in India: A Cultural Psychiatry Retrospective.* Delhi: Motilal Banarsidass Publishers.

Foucault, Michel. 1987. "The Ethic of Care for the Self as a Practice of Freedom: An Interview with Michel Foucault on January 20, 1984." *Philosophy & Social Criticism* 12(2-3): 112–131.

Gadamer, Hans-Georg. 1990. *Wahrheit und Methode: Grundzüge einer philosophischen Hermeneutik.* Tübingen: J. C. B. Mohr.

Geertz, Clifford. 1983. "From the Native's Point of View: On the Nature of Anthropological Knowledge." In *Local Knowledge: Further Essays in Interpretive Anthropology,* ed. Clifford Geertz. New York: Basic Books: 55–70.

Gerow, Edwin. 2000. "India as a Philosophical Problem: McKim Marriott and the Comparative Enterprise." *Journal of the American Oriental Society* 120(3): 410–429.

Halliburton, Murphy. 2004. "Finding a Fit: Psychiatric Pluralism in South India and Its Implications for WHO Studies of Mental Disorder." *Transcultural Psychiatry* 41(1): 80–98.

Halloy, Arnaud, and Vlad Naumescu. 2012. "Learning Spirit Possession: An Introduction." *Ethnos* 77(2): 155–176.

Harris, Grace G. 1989. "Concepts of Individual, Self, and Person in Description and Analysis." *American Anthropologist, New Series* 91(3): 599–612.

Kakar, Sudhir. 1982. *Shamans, Mystics and Doctors: A Psychological Inquiry Into India and Its Healing Traditions.* Boston: Beacon Press.

Lamb, Sarah. 2000. *White Saris and Sweet Mango: Aging, Gender and Body in North India.* Berkeley: University of California Press.

Landfester, Manfred. 2002. "Nietzsches 'Geburt der Tragödie': Antihistorismus und Antiklassizismus zwischen Wissenschaft, Kunst und Philosophie." In *Mehr Dionysos als Apoll: Anitklassizistische Antike-Rezeption um 1900*, ed. Achim Aurnhammer and Thomas Pittrof. Frankfurt: Vittorio Klostermann Verlag.

Luhrmann, Tanya M. 1989. *Persuasions of the Witch's Craft: Ritual Magic and Witchcraft in Present-day England*. Oxford, U.K.: Basil Blackwell.

Luhrmann, Tanya M., Howard Nusbaum, and Ronald Thisted. 2010. "The Absorption Hypothesis: Learning to Hear God in Evangelical Christianity." *American Anthropologist* 112(1): 66–78.

Mahmood, Saba. 2005. *Politics of Piety: The Islamic Revival and the Feminist Subject*. Princeton: Princeton University Press.

———. 2009. "Religious Reason and Secular Affect: An Incommensurable Divide?" *Critical Inquiry: A Voice For Reasoned Inquiry Into Significant Creations Of The Human Spirit* 35(4): 836–864.

Marriott, McKim. 1976. "Hindu Transactions: Diversity Without Dualism." In *Transaction and Meaning: Directions in the Anthropology of Exchange and Symbolic Behaviour*, ed. Bruce Kapferer. Philadelphia: Institute for the Study of Human Issues, 109–142.

———. 1990a. "Constructing an Indian Ethnosociology." In *India through Hindu Categories*, ed. McKim Marriott. New Delhi: Sage Publications, 1–39.

———. 1991. "On 'Constructing an Indian Ethnosociology.'" *Contributions to Indian Sociology* (25): 295–308.

———. 1992. "Alternative Social Sciences." In *General Education in the Social Sciences: Centennial Reflections*, ed. John J. MacAloon. Chicago: University of Chicago Press, 262–278.

———. 1998. "The Female Family Core Explored Ethnosociologically." *Contributions to Indian Sociology* 32(2): 279–304.

———, ed. 1990b. *India through Hindu Categories*. New Delhi: Sage Publications.

Marriott, McKim, and Ronald B. Inden. 1977. "Toward an Ethnosociology of South Asian Caste Systems." In *The New Wind: Changing Identities in South Asia*, ed. Kenneth David. The Hague: Mouton Publishers.

Moffatt, Michael. 1990. "Deconstructing McKim Marriott's Ethnosociology: An Outcast's Critique." *Contributions to Indian Sociology* 24(2): 215–236.

Moore, Melinda. 1990. "The Kerala House as a Hindu Cosmos." In *India through Hindu Categories*, ed. McKim Marriott. New Delhi: Sage Publications, 169–202.

Moreno, Manuel, and McKim Marriott. 1990. "Humoral Transactions in Two Tamil Cults." In *India through Hindu Categories*, ed. McKim Marriott. New Delhi: Sage Publications, 149–167.

Naraindas, Harish. 2006. "Of Spineless Babies and Folic Acid: Evidence and Efficacy in Biomedicine and Ayurvedic Medicine." *Social Science & Medicine* 62 (11): 2658–2669.

———. Forthcoming. "Nosopolitics: Epistemic Mangling and the Creolization of Contemporary Ayurveda." In *Medical Pluralism and Homeopathy in India and Germany (1810-2010): Practices in A Comparative Perspective,* ed. Martin Dinges. Stuttgart: Institute for the History of Medicine, Robert Bosch Stiftung.

Obeyesekere, Gananath. 1990. "The Illusory Pursuit of the Self: A Review of 'Culture and Self: Asian and Western Perspectives' [by Anthony J. Marsella, George DeVos, and Francis L. K. Hsu]." *Philosophy East and West* 40(2): 239–250.

Opler, Morris E. 1958. "Spirit Possession in a Rural Area of North India". In *Reader in Comparative Religion,* ed. William A. Lessa and Evon Vogt. New York: Harper & Row, 553–566.

Osella, Caroline, and Filippo Osella. 2008. "Food, Memory, Community: Kerala as Both 'Indian Ocean' Zone and as Agricultural Homeland." *South Asia: Journal of South Asian Studies* 31(1): 170–198.

Östör, Ákos, and Lina Fruzzetti. 1991. "For an Ethnosociology of India?" *Contributions to Indian Sociology* 25(2): 309–320.

Pakaslahti, Antti. 1998. "Family-centered Treatment of Mental Health Problems at the Balaji Tempel in Rajasthan." In *Changing Patterns of Family and Kinship in South Asia,* ed. Asko Parpola and Sirpa Tenhunen. Helsinki: Studia Orientalia, 129–166.

———. 2005. "Traditional Healers as Culturally Accepted / Sanctioned Mental Health Practitioners." In *Mental Disorders in Children and Adolescents: Need and Strategies for Intervention,* ed. Savita Malhotra. New Delhi: CBS Publishers & Distributors, 215–229.

———. 2008. "Terminology of Spirit Illness: An Empirical Study of a Living Healing Tradition." In *Mathematics and Medicine in Sanskrit,* ed. Dominik Wujastyk. Delhi: Motilal Banarsidass, 155–192.

———. 2009. "Health-Seeking Behavior for Psychiatric Disorders in North India: An Exploration of Medical Pluralism." In *Psychiatrists and Traditional Healers: Unwitting Partners in Global Mental Health,* ed. Mario Incayawar, Ronald Wintrob, and Lise Bouchard. London: Wiley Blackwell, 149–166.

Pfeifer, Samuel. 1994. "Belief in Demons and Exorcism in Psychiatric Patients in Switzerland." *British Journal of Medical Psychology* 67(3): 247–258.

Quack, Johannes. 2010. "Bell, Bourdieu and Wittgenstein on Ritual Sense." In *The Problem of Ritual Efficacy,* ed. William Sax, Johannes Quack, and Jan Weinhold. New York: Oxford University Press, 169–188.

———. 2012a. "Arten des Unglaubens als 'Mentalität': Religionskritische Traditionen in Indien." In *Religion und Kritik in der Moderne,* ed. Ulrich Berner and Johannes Quack. Berlin: LIT-Verlag, 113–138.

———. 2012b. *Disenchanting India: Organized Rationalism and Criticism of Religion in India.* New York: Oxford University Press.

———. 2013. "'What do I know?' Scholastic Fallacies and Pragmatic Religiosity in Mental Health Seeking Behaviour in India." *Mental Health, Religion & Culture* 16(4): 403–418.

Ramanujan, Attipate K. 1990. "Is there an Indian Way of Thinking?" In *India through Hindu Categories,* ed. McKim Marriott. New Delhi: Sage Publications, 41–58.

Rosin, R. Thomas. 2000. "Wind Traffic and Dust: The Recycling of Wastes." *Contributions to Indian Sociology* 34(3): 361–408.

Satija, D. C., S. S. Nathawat, D. Singh, and A. Sharma. 1982. "A Study of Patients Attending Mehandipur Balaji Temple: Psychiatric and Psychodynamic Aspects." *Indian Journal of Psychiatry* 24(4): 375–379.

Sax, William S. 2009. *God of Justice: Ritual Healing and Social Justice in the Central Himalayas*. New York: Oxford University Press.

Sax, William S., and Jan Weinhold. 2010. "Rituals of Possession." In *Ritual Matters. Dynamic Dimensions in Practice,* ed. Ute Hüsken and Christiane Brosius. London: Routledge, 236–252.

Simpson, Bob. 1997. "Possession, Dispossession and the Social Distribution of Knowledge Among Sri Lankan Ritual Specialists." *The Journal of the Royal Anthropological Institute* 3(1): 43–59.

Smith, Frederick M. 2006. *The Self Possessed: Deity and Spirit Possession in South Asian Literature and Civilization*. New York: Columbia University Press.

Spiro, Melford E. 1993. "Is the Western Conception of the Self 'Peculiar' within the Context of the World Cultures?" *Ethos* 21(2): 107–153.

Strathern, Marilyn. 1988. *The Gender of the Gift*. Berkeley: University of California Press.

Taylor, Charles. 1992. *Sources of the Self: Making of the Modern Identity*. Cambridge, U.K.: Cambridge University Press.

———. 1995. "Two Theories of Modernity." *The Hastings Center Report* 25(2): 24–33.

———. 2007. *A Secular Age*. Cambridge, M.A.: The Belknap Press of Harvard University Press.

———. 2008. "Buffered and Porous Selves." *The Immanent Frame*. http://blogs. ssrc.org/tif/2008/09/02/buffered-and-porous-selves. Accessed 3 March 2012.

Uberoi, Jit P. Singh. 1978. *Science and Culture*. Delhi: Oxford University Press.

Whitehouse, Harvey. 2004. *Modes of Religiosity: A Cognitive Theory of Religious Transmission*. Walnut Creek, C.A.: AltaMira Press.

Wrathall, Mark A. 2000. "Background Practices, Capacities and Heideggerian Disclosure." In *Essays in Honor of Hubert L. Dreyfus: Heidegger, Coping, and Cognitive Science,* ed. Hubert L. Dreyfus, Mark A. Wrathall, and John E. Malpas. Cambridge, M.A.: MIT Press, 93–114.

Chapter Three
Medical Individualism and the Dividual Person

Francis Zimmermann

Clinician 7 [medical oncologist]: In Delhi, generally, I can say that from the initial symptom [of breast cancer], to [the presentation of] disease . . . a time factor is something like six months to two to three years . . . Say, some lady has some lump [inside], she will try to take the local help [traditional healer] first. Somebody will say to her, oh no, it will heal automatically; you take this um . . . this local plant . . . Once it's a fungating mass and it's bleeding, oozing pus, something like that, then only they are told that ok this is something that yes, cannot be controlled here.

> —Alex Broom et al., "The Inequalities of Medical Pluralism"

The doctor sensing the anxiety in the couple [consulting for infertility] began by explaining the impact of stress on the endocrinal system.

Dr.: The hypothalamus orders the pituitary to begin its work. FSH and LH [hormones secreted by the pituitary gland] come down to the ovaries where eggs are already present and the FSH and LH stimulate the ovaries and the eggs are matured.

Continuing, she explains the entire process again, this time using an analogy to make it more accessible:

Dr.: . . . if the elders in the family are not good what will the junior or younger people do in such a family? If the family elders set a bad example for the younger lot, what can be expected of the young ones? Look at our country, if our political system is so bad what will become of the country? Same way, the hypothalamus has to set the right example for the pituitary in order for it to be able to stimulate the ovaries. So keep tensions away as it affects the proper functioning of the hypothalamus.

> —Aditya Bharadwaj, "Biosocialities and Biocrossings"

Patients who present with cancer or infertility like the ones mentioned above—among other possible examples since all patients are confronted to the same dichotomy when presenting with any serious complaint—have two basic options for treatment corresponding to two conceptions of themselves and their future. The first option and the most conventional treatments are technologies like in vitro fertilization or chemotherapy. Another option consists of a wide range of alternative therapies, from the use of herbs and nutritional supplements, to psychic therapies, rituals, and meditation. There is an obvious asymmetry between these two basic options. Conventional medicine, backed by extensive studies and statistics, claims to offer the patient the opportunity to know his or her risks before treatment begins, while alternative methods lack the studies and statistics that show success and failure. Therefore, those who choose alternative methods of healing are doing so primarily on faith and are depending on conceptions of life and the human person that support their choice. Working in India, I would like to explore this asymmetry between conventional and alternative options for treatment in the context of medical consultations, admonitions to patients, and other types of conversations or speech acts like the two quotations above. Medical practice has traditionally taken the form of a conversation. Since diagnoses, prognoses, and prescriptions are matters for discourse and dialogue, I am interested in words and concepts formulated in the local language to assess and explain disease.

Language will be the main thread throughout this chapter, and English in the first place, as far as it is used in consultation rooms with educated patients. We shall start from interviews in English. But the description is likely to remain at the surface of things until we turn our attention to language issues and address the potential mistranslations from the local mother-tongue to English and back. All the more so within the framework of the Sanskrit-vernacular diglossia that prevails in India. Ideas such as the self and the other, the mental and the physiological, the causality of disease and the patient's agency, even as they are expressed in English, appear to be modeled on Sanskrit words and phrases in the context of speech events. Consequently, in the course of this chapter we shall be moving from medical discourse in plain English language to the underlying covert Sanskrit categories.

I shall consider situations and therapeutic trajectories in which medical science and local conceptions of health and disease intersect to produce alternative ideologies of the body, the person, natural processes, and human agency. Health and disease will not be taken for granted, in the medical conditions involved; they will be discussed as values and concerns more than as clear-cut facts, when complaints are seemingly medical but more deeply existential since they affect the patient's self-image and his or her conceptions of the body and self, of birth and death, and of humans sharing and transferring vital identities to one another. I shall elaborate on examples of medical conditions like the ones referred to in the foregoing epigraphs, currently occurring on a grand scale in India among the urban middle class with access to advanced biomedical technologies and affluent enough to address whatever scourges have come to be considered as intolerable but at the same time curable. Cancer and infertility, in that respect, might be considered as paradigmatic insofar as in both conditions life and death are at stake.

Let us start from readings on such complaints in India as they are described in the social science literature; the details of practical moves and negotiations involved in the selection of technologies and therapeutic modalities will remain in the background. I am studying concepts and values—more precisely conceptualization processes and value judgments—rather than the patient's itinerary in the health care market. Social science approaches to medicine and the healing traditions of India may be broadly divided into fieldwork research on institutions and practices on the one hand, and discourse analysis on the other. The emphasis hereafter is placed on the latter. I am trying to trace the conceptual genealogies of medical arguments, pondering reasons adduced for therapeutic decisions, exposing presuppositions and citations embedded in medical consultations and teachings. Since only very few examples are given in these pages, I should be explicit about the criteria used for their selection. The medical conditions that I selected for discussion are those of interest to lawyers, philosophers, and theologians, and more generally relevant to medical ethics. Shifting the perspective from social science to medical ethics, we shall consider not exactly how patients conducted their search for a cure or why they complied with such and such therapeutic modalities, but rather which

reasons convincing to them have been adduced or by which philosophical, moral, or religious constraints they considered themselves
to be bound.

Cancer, God's Will, and Infertility

Broom and his colleagues (Tovey and Broom 2007; Broom et al.
2009) have shown that oncology is a suitable site for examining the
interplay of tradition and modernity, economic progress and individual beliefs, and the impact of social inequalities on therapeutic
trajectories in the context of South Asian medical pluralism. Ideas
people in India entertain about cancer and its cure are especially
significant for the following reason. One aspect of cancer peculiar to
India—I am following Broom's argument here—results from the fact
that, in certain social milieus, increased wealth has in turn increased
life expectancy through better standards of living and reduced com-
municable diseases. Cancer has thus shifted from being of limited
importance, in health policy terms, to being a considerable issue with
an aging population. Yet, the majority of the population do not have
access to biomedical cancer facilities, and the more affluent who
do have access bring with them a complex heritage of ideological
constraints. Consequently, in spite of the salient position achieved
by molecular medicine in the treatment of cancer, most patients, as
indicated above in the epigraph, remain under the influence of traditional medicine. Tradition and modernity overlap in their medical
itinerary. Moreover, the syncretism that is described by the sociologist in terms of overlapping therapeutic trajectories can also be ana-
lyzed, as we shall see below, in terms of overlapping scientific and
religious discourses. Cancer may be interpreted as an outcome of
social and environmental circumstances, and therapeutic decision
making can be informed as much by physiological facts as by conceptions of place, community, and identity. Oncology would thus be
one appropriate site to disentangle the complex influences of family
circle and biological environment, the community and the locality,
or technoscientific ideas and religion. A major drawback, however,
in the sociological inquiries conducted by Broom and colleagues has
been to approach TCAM (Traditional, Complementary, and Alternative Medicine), an acronym which in itself is an ethnocentric
phrasing, from the point of view of biomedicine. Favoring TCAM

thus seems to be an act of resistance against biomedicine. As the medical oncologist quoted above unambiguously suggests (when he says "you take this um . . . this local plant . . ."), medicinal plants are prescribed out of ignorance by traditional healers, when the disease is not yet recognized as breast cancer, and when the spontaneous decision of ignoring and bypassing biomedical techniques of diagnosis delays proper treatment until it is too late. From this oncologist's viewpoint, which is adopted by the sociologist, tradition here resists modernity, and choosing alternative modes of treatment (like herbs) amounts to resisting conventional medicine (i.e., chemotherapy); traditional and alternative conceptions of cancer are construed as ways of resisting, bypassing, and circumventing the dominant paradigm of modern oncology. The choice of an alternative is equated with the idea of resistance, and it seems to be a political stance. This interpretation calls for further analysis, however, and I would like to look at the dichotomy between biomedicine and TCAM from a different angle.

On a superficial level of analysis, the dichotomy is that of two spheres of life, a mere sociological division. "Alternative medicines are ingrained in our social and cultural system," another clinician says. "Even, you see, at home, if you have some abdominal discomfort or headache, you don't go to a doctor, they'll say 'try some home remedies.' Even your elders within the family will give you some medicines, or they'll go, take you to the Homeopath or Ayurvedic, or some practitioner." For these clinicians "being Indian" necessarily involves use of traditional practices, at least to treat ordinary ailments. Traditional medicine is part of their education within the community. Not surprisingly, each of the clinicians interviewed had personally used TCAM for minor complaints (colds or cuts and bruises) and the response "of course I use them" was typical. "We tell our cancer patients not to use them and then we go home and use them ourselves." Allegiances are split between home and work; the "everyday" nature of use of TCAM and its integral role in Indian sensibilities and the home environment contrast with the preeminence of modern science in the workplace. Broom speaks of ambivalence, disjunction, dichotomy; however, the medical professionals themselves are committed to tradition as part of their everyday lives, while concurrently serving as strong advocates for the validity of modern values and scientific rationality in their professional activity.

Is there more to this division of labor than an ideological divide between traditional ways and modern values? Broom suggests another interpretation in discussing entitlements to treatment, when he mentions prejudices based on gender and inequalities that condemn women suffering from breast cancer to turn to biomedicine when it is too late. Often the fatal delay that prevents women from consulting cancer clinicians early enough results from family elders deciding that females are a low priority in terms of using expensive technologies. In a "patriarchal" society, as Broom says, it is apparently all right for women to take the risk of TCAM while males, whose earnings are essential to the family, are so precious as to justify spending resources for their treatment in modern facilities. Women, for whom traditional therapies are good enough, are left in the hands of God, so to say. This inequality in entitlements represents the utilitarian side of a religious worldview. A worldview wherein what is most valuable is the perpetuation and welfare of the family, not of individuals. The target to meet, in providing the best medical care available to males, is not saving the life *of individuals* in the family, but saving the life *of the family* beyond all individual deaths. The family elders who decide who will be given which kind of treatment seem to adopt a double standard that entails a dichotomy between technical rationality for the individual's sake and religious rationality for the sake of the community. This is endorsed by clinicians themselves. While maintaining a theoretical distinction of rationality/accountability as delineating biomedical cancer care from TCAM, despite the rational/metaphysical dichotomy evident initially in their accounts, a few clinicians cited by Broom were in the habit of contextualizing failures in treatment and their own perceived "failings" (whenever they feel lack of certainty, consistency, technologies, or mastery) by placing success and failure within a metaphysical framework and comforting the patient with sayings such as "God willing" or "It is up to the gods." A "clinical theodicy," if we may borrow the phrase from a brilliant paper by Aditya Bharadwaj (2008), who heard this kind of justificatory discourse uttered by clinicians engaged in infertility medicine, comes to be superimposed upon clinical rationality.

A theodicy is invented to give meaning to suffering and to mitigate frustration when rational explanations in terms of empirical causation fail to justify human suffering or misfortune. Religious beliefs are adduced as coping mechanisms for the clinicians and their patients as they struggle to make sense of intractable conditions. This is a fairly common discourse among biomedical clinicians, although not so explicit in oncology as when applied to success and failure of in vitro fertilization, a technology that by its very nature problematizes cultural understandings of birth and fate; metaphysical tenets are invoked to justify treatment outcomes and limitations in both domains as well. Following Bharadwaj, Broom and his colleagues suggested that this attitude or mode of thought, whenever observed in modern medical settings, was borrowed from TCAM. They pointed to an internal tension, in medical domains they explored as sociologists in South Asia, between individual interests and rationality on the one side since biomedicine in principle treats an individual patient, and community and religious beliefs on the other side.

One suspects, however, that inquiries proceeding by interviews will remain at the surface of things until we turn our attention to language and verbal performance in medical consultations. Utterances and statements, in the course of medical encounters between patients and doctors—or clinicians or practitioners or healers or whatever they are to be called—that are supposed to convey the different ideologies of health and disease to be compared, should be contextualized from the angle of addressivity. Addressivity (in linguistic terminology) is the quality of turning to someone in the course of a conversation involving more than two participants. It is a well-known medical sociological observation that, whenever there are more than two individuals present in the consultation room because the patient is accompanied by family members or because the senior clinician is assisted by his juniors and nurses, the doctor may seem to overtly speak to the patient while, actually but covertly, his assistants or the patient's family members are the real addressees. The doctor addresses his comments to those who can answer, give sanction to, or assume responsibility for choices to be made. Addressivity focuses attention on the medical trajectory assigned to the patient with her consent or not, depending on her individual answerability, standing, and entitlements. But of course in the advent of medical ethics the rights of the individual patient have progressively been recognized. I would like to suggest that, from the angle of addressivity alone, there is already a significant difference between modern medicine, which has come to respect individual consent and to favor face-to-face encounter, and traditional practice still attached to family and community values. When the clinician recommends chemotherapy by saying: "Statistics indicate x percent success and, in your case, the prospects are good," this utterance is addressed to the individual patient who is free to decide. To the contrary, addressees of the traditional practitioner's utterances and prescriptions are in most cases those in authority at the family or even the community level. A notable exception occurs when a dedicated doctor like Mahadeva Iyer—whose demeanor will be discussed in the last section below—out of his sense of a bond of nature between all creatures, endeavors to systematically establish a one-to-one relationship with patients.

But there is more to language than this play on overt and covert addressivity. Disease, in traditional discourse, is not a clear-cut complaint to be easily objectified under a penetrating clinical gaze, but an equivocal, multifaceted condition in which different levels of reality are superimposed on one another. It is through naming and categorizing these levels of reality in Sanskrit that Ayurvedic doctors decipher the patient's physiology cum personality as if it were a palimpsest. Due to the ubiquitous Sanskrit-vernacular diglossia, medical knowledge and discourse are grounded on a mixed language which locally constitutes the mother-tongue of educated people. We might like to retrieve the mother-tongue version of all statements in English quoted in the sociological literature I have been using, in order to assess the faithfulness of translations.

To anyone familiar with South Asian philosophies, there is a misunderstanding on the English name of God when it is pronounced in the context of medical consultations in India. All the more so since a phrase like "God willing" in English is one of several key rhetorical practices used as markers of alternative ideologies of medicine as when an informant emphasizes the rational/metaphysical dichotomy in the following way:

> Clinician 14 [pediatric hematologist]: Even today, even in these . . . alternative [Ayurveda, homeopathy, Unani] . . . when traditional practitioners talk, they talk in superlatives. When I talk, I say [for example], the cure rate is seventy percent . . . The traditional practitioners, he [sic] says, "don't worry, it will be all right. I'll give you courage and God willing, you will be all right, you know" . . . that word "God willing" . . . gives [him] an easy way out. (Broom et al. 2009: 701)

In other words, the hematologist quotes statistics while the traditional practitioner invokes God. But the name of God in medical contexts calls for a gloss to expose the rationale behind the usage. The student of Sanskrit medical texts cannot fail to note that the English phrases—*God willing* and *It is up to the gods*—here translate an Ayurvedic principle that is part of the classical doctrine of therapeutic prognosis, the structure of which is very different from our own Western scheme. Ayurvedic doctors make use of a triadic division of the causes of success or failure in medical treatment. If and when a treatment achieves healing, this success in cure results from a specific balance among three different principles of causality and three different types of cure. The doctrine of three causalities is taught in the *Carakasaṃhitā*, Sūtra 11.54 and Vimāna 8.87:

1. The first causes of successful cure are *daivavyapāśraya*, that is, those "placed in [the hands of] gods *(daiva)*," or "based on fate *(daiva)*," and "It is up to the gods" is a cut-and-dried phrase referring to the causality of destiny.
2. The second causes of success are *yuktivyapāśraya*, "based on reasoning," or more exactly on the physician's clever "manipulation of conjunctions" *(yukti)* between the patient's body and her environment.
3. The third causes of success result from the patient's "willpower" *(sattvāvajaya)*.

It would take too long to develop in all textual detail the philosophical arguments underlying this triadic division, which takes different forms in medicine and in other branches of learning. I shall limit myself to saying that it entails a threefold classification of traditional sciences, when it is said that there are three disciplines useful for curing diseases in ailing humans, namely, Medicine (establishing proper junctions between the body and environment), Grammar (the rules for the accurate recitation and transmission of the Word on things divine), and Yoga (strengthening our mental powers). This classification corresponds term-to-term to the triadic division of the causes of disease. The first type of cause of disease is the inappropriate conjunction between our sense organs and their objects *(asātmyendriyārtha)*; medical reasoning *(yukti)* is the art of restoring congruent conjunctions. The second type of cause is breaches of wisdom *(prajñāparādha)*, for which the appropriate therapy is willpower and discipline of the self. The third mode of disease causality is fate (*pariṇāma*), and any therapeutic action to be resorted to in that respect falls in the realm of religious institutions and practices. In the face of this classical doctrine, Broom's dichotomy between the rational, that would characterize conventional medicine, and the metaphysical, that would characterize traditional and alternative ideologies of health and disease, does not hold. There is no fixed dichotomy, but a context-sensitive combination of three dimensions. Furthermore, we should not fall victims to the spiritualistic connotations that are falsely introduced in the biased translation of Sanskrit *daivavyapāśraya* into English "God willing," or "It is up to the gods." It is true that *daiva* means either "the gods" or "fate, destiny," but this word and concept clearly belongs with the physical dimension of the world, and not the spiritual, as will be shown below.

Let us go back over what we called a *clinical theodicy* invented by oncologists to justify failures in treatment by placing success and failure "in the hands of God." The social scientists I was quoting above suggested that this justificatory discourse was imported from traditional medicine. There might be some truth to this suggestion as far as the comparison of the English phrases involved with Sanskrit *daivavyapāśraya* makes sense, but a precise reading of the Sanskrit texts, as we have seen, reveals a misunderstanding since the Ayurvedic doctrine of the three *causalities of disease* is definitely not justificatory. We are faced here with a completely different mode of thought. Disease, in South Asian classical teachings, is not a well-delineated complaint that can be ascertained by anatomical/pathological diagnosis, but a mixed condition produced by the superimposition of different levels of reality in the patient's body. From a cosmological viewpoint, the doctrine of the three causes of health and disease entails a tridimensional conception of life in this world, a doctrine that was shared by several ancient Indian and Greek philosophical schools. This triadic division has been retrieved in contemporary anthropology as shown in the following formulation inspired by McKim Marriott (1990), to which I shall later return:

1. A first dimension, *the physical dimension,* is that of mixing (absorption, rebirth) versus unmixing (subtraction, death); this is "fate" (*daiva*), or the time dimension;

2. Another dimension, *the ethical dimension,* is that of unmarking versus marking; this is human agency, or "willpower" (*sattva*) materialized as a fluid in the body channels, better understood as the function or activity of taking decisions;
3. The third analytic dimension, *the logical dimension,* is that of unmatching (disorder) versus matching (order); this is the realm of human "reasoning" (*yukti*), or the art of congruent "junctions" (*yoga*).

The relative importance of each of the three dimensions for a given medical condition varies according to context and can only be assessed in the context of a particular case history.

Let us pause for a moment and reflect upon the nature of the materials dealt with here. This is mainstream discourse currently held by all learned Ayurvedic physicians in India on the causality of disease, the patient's agency, and the seasoned doctor's well-balanced prescriptions, since they studied the relevant classic texts in medical school. Our vital lead in our analysis is a set of Sanskrit words—*daiva, sattva,* and *yukti*—that represent three major categories of thought ethnographically significant in South Asia. These are local categories, that is, concepts and values phrased in the local language, that come to the forefront in the context of speech events, be it in the classroom or in the consultation room. All important Sanskrit terms and phrases are locally embedded in the vernacular (Hindi, Malayalam, etc.). This approach to the Ayurvedic medical discourse in terms of performance will be elaborated upon in the second part of this contribution when we shall study grids, lists, and schemes to be applied in specific contexts.

A final remark is in order on the first of the foregoing dimensions which is sometimes mistranslated, as we have seen, into God's will. One should emphasize the fact that the triad of *daiva, sattva,* and *yukti* is devoid of any spiritual or spiritualistic connotations. There are domains of medicine like infertility medicine or transplants where the *daiva* plane and the alternation of birth and death play an essential role.

Infertility medicine, in that respect, is a domain still more relevant and topical than oncology, because medicine there is even more constrained by social values and philosophical presuppositions, namely, the treatment of nonbirth. Bharadwaj (2006) has shown that the transfer to India of in vitro fertilization (IVF) initiated new modes of reasoning whenever the success or failure of assisted conception, as explained by clinicians to infertile consumers, was situated in the universe of Hindu faith. Technologies of procreation like IVF are not transferred into cultural voids. In the context of a clinician's faith, assisted conception juxtaposes tradition and modernity, science and religion, social values in this world like family relationships and the laws of biology. The clinical engagement with infertility and the patient's choice in favor of assisted conception provide an insight into how people simultaneously inhabit several domains. The clinician quoted at the outset of this chapter, who, in the course of an infertility consultation, draws an analogy between the influence of the hypothalamus over the pituitary and the influence of family elders over the young couple, provides a clear example of such a juxtaposition. This pedagogical analogy will be convincing to the patient only because the 24-year-old young wife, who anxiously wants a child, lives under a dramatic social constraint, stigmatized as she is by the overweening patriarchal expectations of her in-laws, who fault her for infertility. The clinician's discourse strikingly suggests a linkage between social and biological constraints that Bharadwaj (2008) describes under the name of *biosocialities*. But one should also remember that stigma and the medicalization of infertility here are situated in the context of Hinduism. Bharadwaj invites attention to two intersecting domains: on the one side, Hindu cosmology that produces beliefs and norms about human fertility or infertility, which in turn produce the experience of stigma and social suffering in the face of infertility; and, on the other side, the modern institution of biomedicine, which is indigenized by its location in the wider context of Hindu traditions. Parallel or complementary to Bharadwaj, who focuses on the latter to show how technoscientific ideas have been reformulated, one can put the emphasis on the tradition side and point to indigenous institutions or representations that prefigure the foregoing conflation between social relationships and biological identities.

The South Asian *joint family* is one such institution, the analysis of which will help us shift from sociological aspects of medical intervention to cosmologies and representations. In Bharadwaj's field interviews of husbands (28 percent), wives (21 percent), and couples (46 percent) that have been frequenting clinics specializing in IVF,[1] one significant figure is that 60.5 percent of the interviewed treatment seekers, all Hindus, described their family arrangement as "joint" while 39.5 percent described themselves as living in a nuclear family (Bharadwaj 2003: 1869). The joint family is as much a socio-logical fact as a set of moral and religious representations. A Hindu joint or undivided family consists of at least three generations living together under one roof, sharing the same kitchen, with a common place of worship. Descent or filiation is given more importance than marital ties, and the joint family is structured around a core set of three kinship positions, namely, those of brother, sister, and nephew. We should never forget the structural fact that, in order for the joint family to perpetuate itself, women should be given in marriage by their father or brother to their in-laws, and that their male child, the brother's nephew, is the offspring par excellence since he will remain under the same roof and participate in the perpetuation of the undivided family. The South Asian kinship triad of brother/sis-ter/nephew in which descent overlaps with marriage is one of the complex social and biological ideas underpinning attitudes toward the birth or nonbirth of a child, because in the institution and rep-resentation of the joint family the corporeal connection between the married couple and their offspring is at once biological (the child is their offspring) and social (the child is the niece or nephew of some elder in authority). Therefore we must carefully avoid misrepresen-tations when describing the two triads to be considered in medi-cal situations studied by Bharadwaj, although he was perspicacious enough to notice (2003: 1870) that *"the invisible biological triangle"* of womb, semen, and fetus underscores *"the socially visible triad"* of parents and offspring. In the context of the South Asian joint fam-ily, it does not make much sense to define in Bharadwaj's terms the socially visible triad as that of "mother, father and child" (Bharadwaj 2003: 1870), as if the young couple and their offspring constituted an independent social monad, while it would be accurate and quite illuminating to say that the biological triad of womb, semen, and fetus underscores the social triad of sister, brother, and nephew. What is eagerly desired in an infertile couple's missing child, in the context of South Asian values and for the family to thrive, is not simply a baby but an offspring—structurally speaking, a nephew—who will both assume transmission of the family estate and alliance between his kin and their in-laws. Whenever infertility is stigmatized in Hindu milieus studied by Bharadwaj, it is because people resent being deprived of a nephew to perpetuate the family. This phrasing of the relationship between the biological and the social is free of any individualistic overtones, and facilitates alternative approaches to disease and medicine in terms of transactions and performances.

Triads, Quartets, and Other Dividualities

The sociologists and anthropologists cited in the first part chose to remain within the framework of contemporary Westernized clinical settings, where interactions between biomedicine and TCAM take the form of a dialectic between domination and resistance. These two concepts have been, since the early 1980s, the received wisdom of medical anthropologists who have shown how people (individual patients, families, or even sects and shrines in India) resist dominant cultural paradigms of health. "Empower the patient," so that she would be capable to bypass the dominant ideologies of health and the conventional modes of medical care; that was the motto. Observers describing the institutions of TCAM downplayed the role of the healer's competence and favored the performance of healing, I mean the politics of medicine. The fact that forms of TCAM were knowledge systems worth studying for themselves was taken for granted. I would like to reverse the perspective and consider alternative institutions and practices insofar as they are based on knowledge systems.

Let us then shift gears, turn our attention to South Asian languages and concepts, and take two steps toward a different epistemology. First, I would like to start from Sanskrit categories, as we did already when substituting the Western division between "the rational and the metaphysical" with the triad of *daiva* (fate), *yukti* (reasoning), and *sattva* (willpower). A welcome discovery, when shifting languages, is that South Asian categories seem able to simultaneously represent modes of thought (religious, rational, and moral) on the one hand and physical realities (fate, conjunctions, and agency) on the other hand, whereas English ones could not. Second, indigenous categories are context-sensitive; they summarize our lived experience in a given cultural and historical milieu, and starting from Sanskrit categories will help to articulate knowledge with practice. This analysis is only concerned with Ayurvedic medicine because of my limitations, but on the other hand very few social scientists have access to the Sanskrit texts underlying practice, while in my own work I have always proceeded from readings in medical Sanskrit to field observations in Ayurvedic clinics. Indian pandits and learned *vaidyas* (traditional practitioners) have developed and laid down in the classic texts a panoply of triads and quartets—like the three humors, the four human pursuits—and other grids and schemata which all represent keys for experience, performance, and action. We should study them from inside. I shall follow McKim Marriott's multidimensional analysis of Hindu categories (1990) and I shall select examples relevant to health, disease, and medicine. Examples are easy to find since the medical discourse of traditional practitioners, in the texts as well as in consultation rooms and the clinic, is peppered with the recitation of stereotyped series of items.

The difficulty in studying medical traditions is that Indologists are accustomed to remain at the level of denotational textuality, juggling with Sanskrit words and citations without taking into account the performance of practice—emotions, gestures, dialogues, and demeanor. But to repeat the leitmotif marking out successive turning points in the course of this analysis, concepts and values must be set back in the context of practice, because Sanskrit phrases are keys for action. For example the doctor abruptly says to the addressee (not necessarily the patient, as we have seen, but the patient's family members or the doctor's assistant): *tan mehān piṭakāviṣam,* and this elliptic and formulaic utterance, an octosyllabic quarter of a distich meaning "This [ghee cures all forms of] diabetes [with] boils and [blood] poisoning," suffices to settle the diagnosis and prescribe the treatment. It may be a pointed utterance addressed to someone who will recognize here a fragment of the celebrated *Dhanvantara-ghṛtayoga,* the "recipe" (*yoga*) of a medicated ghee recommended for all forms of diabetes (*prameha*) with complications like boils (*piṭakā*) and blood poisoning (*viṣa*). Or it may be, so to say, a baited utterance addressed to no one in particular so that the listeners who understand this Sanskrit phrase will pick up what is to be done next—i.e., booking the diabetic patient in a twenty-one-day course of *pañca-karma* treatment including potions of Dhanvantari Ghee—while the listeners who do not catch the meaning will nevertheless take the bait and respectfully ask for a gloss in the vernacular giving them the diagnosis and the prescription. This is the way Sanskrit words here operate as keys for action.

I would even like to expand the notion of performance to the classic texts when cited in any given public context. An illustration of the performative value of medical citations from Sanskrit or vernaculars like Tamil is to be found in an institution recently created to ensure legal protection of intellectual property rights over medicinal plant properties in the pharmaceutical industry. Since the 1980s, transnational corporations have tried to patent allegedly new medicines that are actually modeled on traditional formulas, and the TCAM establishment in India riposted by compiling and digitizing the TKDL (Traditional Knowledge Database Library), a gigantic repository of triads, quartets, and other lists of items in Sanskrit and the vernaculars, which are successfully produced in court to challenge improper patent applications.[2] Citation is action. This is why we may speak of the performative value of yogas (versified recipes) retrieved from the TKDL, whenever they are produced to document the preexistence of traditional knowledge and counteract unwelcome patent applications. Since the quotation of a given Sanskrit recipe prevails against foreign attempts at isolating some of its ingredients, patenting them, and manufacturing the "new" pharmaceutical on an industrial scale, we may conclude that the antique formulas do retain their performative value in the age of technological reproducibility, as Walter Benjamin would have put it.

The impact of language and linguistic processes like *lexicalization* and *diglossia* on traditional practice cannot be overestimated. The contemporary language shift to English in India has created the illusion that the art of diagnosis, prescriptions, and Ayurvedic pharmaceuticals have remained the same when traditional *vaidyas* began to study and practice Ayurvedic medicine in English. This illusion is reinforced by the fact that the older diglossia, in which Sanskrit was superimposed to the local vernacular, was substituted with a newer one in which English replaced Sanskrit. But the older mode of thought was lost in translation, because the new doctor did not make use of citations and formulaic utterances any more. Citation was action in the traditional clinic itself. One might like to qualify this statement but, broadly speaking and as far as traditional Ayurvedic practice was concerned, there was no place for narratives.[3] Observations on the medical constitution and complaints of individual patients, diagnosis, and therapeutic prescriptions were made in the form of stereotyped phrases based upon lists of categories like the three *doṣas*. A well-trained practitioner was able to juggle multiple occurrences of one and the same category in different lists and the multiple synonyms of one and the same name; physiological or pharmaceutical correlations and synergies were brought to the fore whenever two or more occurrences or synonyms of a given word were mentioned in the performance of practice.

This kind of pragmatics might take place in any language including English, provided that the medical consultation is not limited to a face-to-face encounter with the individual patient but involves other listeners ready to catch the illocutory effects of medical utterances phrased in a specific terminology. But what is highly specific to Ayurvedic discourse is its dividual orientation, that is, the propensity to divide all categories into their multiple facets, beginning with the patient's self. Our next step, in tfhe second half of this chapter, will be to transpose the scheme of multifaceted categories at large to the dividual person of the patient in particular.

One last clue to the discovery of this dividual orientation in South Asian local knowledge is the mechanism of synonymity in Sanskrit nomenclatures and the process of lexicalization on which it is based. One and the same item is given several names that represent as many facets of this item. The *Carakasaṃhitā*, Sūtra 4.22, reads: *"eko'pi hy anekāṃ saṃjñāṃ labhate kāryāntarāṇi kurvan"* (One and the same practitioner gets hold of the plurality of names when performing different actions). In other words, nomenclatures are elaborated in performance. A medieval Sanskrit commentary gives the following explanation:

> One and the same person while performing different acts gets different names (*saṃjñā*) by virtue of his position and association with the acts performed or the means adopted for such performance, and a nomenclature of occupations is created thus: one who cooks is a *cook*, one who makes pots is a *potter*, one who digs the earth with a shovel is a *shoveler*, etc. Likewise, one and the same drug entering in different compounds to cure different diseases gets different names in different contexts, and a nomenclature of medicinal properties is created thus: the *kṣīrakākolī* for example (a tuberous root) is alternatively designated by nouns (*saṃjñā*) such as *Roborative, Nourishing, Spermatogenic*, etc.

These are no longer treated as adjectives, they are lexicalized as it were and treated as nouns and synonyms of *kṣīrakākolī*. A discussion

101

of the problematics of naming and of the concept of *saṃjñā* in the Hindu and Buddhist traditions of India would fall beyond the scope of the present chapter, and I can only say here that categories— when speaking of *doṣas* (the three humors of Ayurvedic medicine) as categories for example—are nouns or *saṃjñās*. Categories are created in Sanskrit through a process of lexicalization taking place in the course of performing an action, and reciprocally, triads, quartets, and other fixed lists of categories illustrate the propensity of pundits for facet design and dividual modes of thought.

In learned forms of Ayurvedic practice until some decades ago, the doctor's diagnoses and prescriptions were collectively addressed to the patient and any witness to the consultation in the vernacular language—Malayalam for example when I did fieldwork in Kerala— with a number of Sanskrit citations embedded in the conversation and stereotyped utterances referring to different lists of three, four, five, or six or seven or twenty categories to be taken into account. Contrary to the patient-centered approach and the mode of face-to-face communication between the doctor and the patient that have become prevalent in modern culture, the plurality of addressees attending the Ayurvedic consultation and the fragmentation of medical conversation into fixed phrases and lists of items emphasized the dependency of the individual patient on her family circle. The patient was sometimes reduced to dumbness if not even to the position of a *nonperson* in Erving Goffman's sense of the word, her individuality dissolved as it were into the anonymity of humors and complaints. The whole medical performance perfectly illustrated Marriott's assertion that, in South Asian ethnosociology, "persons are composite and divisible (what one might better call 'dividuals') and that interpersonal relations in the world are generally irregular and fluid, if not entirely chaotic" (1990: 17). The most convincing evidence was produced in the multiple ways that the word *doṣa* was used. The *doṣas* are the most salient features of Hindu medical discourse, located at the point of intersection between different overlapping series. *Doṣas* are of two types: *vātādi* and *rāgādi*. Rather than being "morbific entities" or "faulty conditions" (to mention two current translations), the *doṣas* are fluids, three of them (the *vātādi* series—wind, bile, and phlegm) distributed all over the body, and six more (the series of passions or *rāgādi* series—desire, hate, avarice, etc.) concentrated in the heart. But again the *rāgādi-doṣas* are included in the list of adventitious faulty conditions that comprises traumas "like possession, etc." (*bhūtādi*) and passions "like desire, etc." (*rāgādi*), and again they are included in the body-mind division of diseases, when the list of organic diseases "like fever, etc." (*jvarādi*) is opposed to the list of mental diseases "like desire, etc." (*rāgādi*). This outline of humoral combinatorics relies on an important presupposition: one must never forget that all these various *doṣas* are fluids. A translation favoring the adjectival content of Ayurvedic categories, as when *doṣas* are construed as morbific entities, tends to misrepresent their physiological reality; categories are nouns designating constituents of a composite, divisible, and reticulated reality, just as *doṣas* as fluid constituents of a living being's physiology.

A feature common to all Hindu lists of categories is "that moral and physical are mutually translatable" (Marriott 1990: 7). Physical phenomena like wind, fire, and water appear in the lists on an equal footing with human moral qualities and psychological states like willpower and desire. They seem to represent different facets of one and the same psychophysical reality. The intertwining of the moral and the physical is highlighted in the most recent presentations of Ayurvedic treatments like *śirodhārā*—which consists of gently bathing the head with a flow (*dhārā*) of medicated oil—to alleviate hemiplegia. In the following advertisement retrieved from the website of an elegant health resort in Kovalam (Kerala, South India),[4] readers should compare the narrative style of the first paragraph describing a cerebrovascular accident occurring in the *brain* (repeated four times) to the discursive style of the second paragraph subtly blending therapeutic effects on the *mind* and the body's *energy balance* with physiological processes of blood supply, blood vessels, blood pressure, and the *circulatory system* (italics are mine to underline specific words and redundancies):

> Stroke is the term used to describe a sudden loss of function in a portion of the *brain*. Typically, that loss of function results in difficulty in moving an arm or leg (paralysis). There may be loss of feeling or peculiar sensations in the same areas. Stroke may also appear with problems relating to sudden loss of speech, blurred vision, and unconsciousness or as a convulsion. The loss of *brain* function is due to a sudden reduction of the blood supply to a portion of the *brain*. The reduced blood supply may be due to clogging of the blood vessel by thickening and hardening of vessel wall or rupture of the blood vessel. Once started, a stroke can

continue to damage the *brain* either by clotting an obstruction or by further hemorrhage.

At Vasudeva Ayurvedic Health Resort, our experienced Ayurvedic physicians give effective treatment for stroke. Physiotherapy along with herbal medications can *lessen the symptoms* of stroke. Body massages help in preventing the inactive muscles from degenerating and the herbal medicines help in stimulating the *circulatory system*. Powerful ayurvedic oils and herbal medicines are used for this. Health is maintained in an individual when the vital *energy* is kept *balanced* throughout one's body. Panchakarma helps to keep arteries healthy and also to keep up normal blood pressure. Exercises are also prescribed according to the condition of the patient. Ayurvedic therapies normalize the body's *energy balance* and help in improving the *circulatory system*. This treatment works strongly on the *mind* as well and induces relaxation, thus *reducing the symptoms* of stroke.

The argument remains entirely within the realm of a Westernized discourse on the benefits of physiotherapy (massages), herbal medicines, and *pañcakarma* resorted to as a symptomatic treatment ("reducing the symptoms"), without giving any clue to the real nature of the vital energy whose balance should be normalized by Ayurvedic therapies. Just a remark in passing on the word *pañcakarma* which functions here as bait. To patients who ask what this exotic Sanskrit word means, the doctor will answer that it is a set of special treatments like *śirodhārā* that were invented by Kerala physicians and confidentially transmitted to their disciples. Actually, the doctor will play on the ambiguous connection of this piece of local and practical knowledge with the classical scheme of *pañcakarma* designating scheduled courses of treatment by evacuants (like laxatives) mitigated with oil baths for seven, fourteen, or twenty-one days in a nursing home. The classical scheme is turned around to suit the modern paradigm of physiotherapy. This is a clear case of intellectual dependency in which English words like *brain* and *circulatory system* seem to provide the accurate and precise meaning of fuzzy notions like mental equipoise and energy balance. Ayurveda and biomedicine reinforce each other in a loop, as it were, since traditional humoralism is turned around to reconcile with the description of a cerebrovascular disease.

In the Ayurvedic chart of the body, there is a fluid controlling the circulation of all the other fluids in the vessels, which sets in motion and distributes the various forms of energy like the nervous impulse, and which is responsible for the balance or imbalance of all the other factors of physiology. This is *vāta*, the humor "wind," and hemiplegia resulting from a stroke like all other neurological diseases is a *vāta* disease. To be more precise, the scheme underlying the prescription of *śirodhārā* in the foregoing example is a twofold scheme. First, the gentle pouring of tepid medicated oil on the patient's scalp and forehead works against obstruction and paralysis that are forms of marking for which *kapha* (phlegm) is responsible; clarifying mind and blood, the oil bath regulates *kapha*. Then, the core pharmacody-namic action of medicated oils works toward matching and continu-ity in physiological processes, alleviation of all forms of unmatching for which *vāta* is responsible.

Language Categories and Individuation

At this point, another methodological shift is required to do alter-native and traditional medicine full justice. One may criticize the fact that we have been using Sanskrit words and their conventional translations, like "wind" and "phlegm" for *vāta* and *kapha,* which inevitably blur the description of clinical cases and physiological processes by peppering actual cases and processes with queer and exotic connotations. Scholars of Ayurveda tend to divide themselves between those who keep dozens of Sanskrit words untranslated and those who have recourse to conventional translations. In both cases, one acknowledges the fact that key words in Ayurveda consti-tute an analytic language of its own that is a true alternative to the terminologies of biomedicine. However, neither of these two solu-tions is satisfactory, because the continuous enunciation of Sanskrit words is bound to drown the Ayurvedic discourse in exoticism if not even in mystery while conventional translations, because they keep close to the primary meaning of the Sanskrit word, convey fancy and potentially ridiculous images of animal spirits blowing in, and mucus oozing out, of the body channels. Let us be aware of the difference between a word like *vāta,* an image like wind blowing in a pipe, and a concept like order-and-disorder, or matching-and-un-matching. (Incidentally, the fact that a pair of contraries like order and disorder, or matching and unmatching, constitute one and the same concept, has been known in the West since Plato and in India since the Upanishads.) Sanskrit words are treacherous things to any

105

addressee in modern parlance since they call to mind vivid images of physical objects or movements. It is difficult to unravel the intricate syndrome of images and concepts in one of those key words like *doṣa* or *vāta* that, following Durkheim and Mauss, we used to call "thought and language categories" (*catégories de pensée et de langue*). Therefore, it is necessary to pay the utmost attention to the original phrasing, the grammar, lexicon, and figures of speech, and to the subtle interplay between images and concepts, if we want to avoid getting tangled up in Sanskrit exoticism and fancy connotations. Let us come back to the foregoing advertisement for oil baths at Vasudeva Ayurvedic Health Resort and reflect upon this particular example. Insofar as we would like to underscore the rationale and logic of *śirodhārā* without getting tangled up in ambiguous imagery of phlegm and wind, we must focus on processes and processual variables such as marking (obstructing) and unmarking (clarifying), or matching (conjoining) and unmatching (disordering), that are at work in living beings. The temperament of a given patient is comprised of the three postulations (*tridoṣa*) of mixing (*pitta*), marking (*kapha*), and unmatching (*vāta*) in specific proportions. The gentle pouring of tepid medicated oil on the head and forehead to alleviate the symptoms of stroke, when applying *śirodhārā*, works against marking (obstruction, paralysis) and toward matching (articulation); beneath the imagery of phlegm causing obstruction and wind causing disarticulation, a double process *against marking and toward matching* is initiated—this is the conceptual content of Ayurvedic teachings in this particular case.

I am not considering here the doctrinal tenets of Ayurveda as a system, but reflecting upon particular medical cases and situations observed in South Asian urban settings, where there is an ongoing competition among different medical paradigms, where individualism is a social value, and where some freedom of interpretation is left to the educated patient, who is making choices among different therapeutical methods as well as coping with ideological and institutional constraints which only make sense insofar as patients construe them as constitutive of their specific lived world. This approach is inspired by Marriott's ethnosociological model of the South Asian "dividual person" introduced in the 1970s. Leaving aside the more recent literature as well as all developments on the Self and the Other in contemporary philosophy of mind, which will remain on the horizon, I shall limit myself here to a brief presentation of the South Asian traditional concepts of multiple selves and living bodies in medicine, their impact on medical ethics and the principle of friendliness with the other recognized as both the same as, and different from, the self beyond the death or the skin of an individual patient (her death and her skin representing two sorts of boundaries for a human individual). I am interested in the Hindu and Buddhist principle of individuation, which is, as is well known, a principle of fragmentation. Individuation is the process by which individuals become differentiated from one another. Hindus and Buddhists think that this world of lived experience, illusory as it may be, is the product of such a fragmentation. Before the human being comes onto the scene, there are no individuals. It is the human being that, in its very effort to know anything, objectifies an appearance for itself that involves the fragmentation of the lived world and its breakup into a display of individuals and of dialogical performances among them on the social scene.

Language is essential to world making through Hindu categories, although, as far as I know, the tools of sociolinguistics and semiotics have unfortunately never been applied to the study of categories—neither in Europe after Durkheim and Mauss nor in America after Sapir and Whorf. Nevertheless, Marriott's ethnosociological enterprise relied upon the implicit recognition of the central position of verbal interaction in South Asian institutions and practices, since categories are words meant to be enunciated by speakers expressing thought for action, as when an Ayurvedic doctor uses Sanskrit words to formulate a diagnosis, a prognosis, and a prescription for the benefit of an individual patient or any other addressees, as explained in a previous section of this chapter. Thought and language categories are words that motivate the speaker to perform what they say. Hindu categories, insofar as they are specific to Sanskrit and the Hindu learned traditions, represent at the same time universal constituent processes in this particular worldview and utterances by which individuals interacting with one another make postulations. In his introductory chapter to *India through Hindu Categories,* Marriott emphasized the transactional aspect of categories, calling them "transactional concepts," but their dialogical aspect also should not be overlooked. In retrospect, one might say that, in the 1970s, when transactionalism pervaded all social sciences, combinatorics was in the foreground to the detriment of linguistics. Marriott defined categories as processual variables or relational properties bound to relate and compare with one another, to exchange and shift positions. But one should not downplay the fact that, in medical matters to say the least, all medical transactions occur in the context of speech events, which in turn entails the fact that, in medical discourse to say the least, set patterns of words are an essential feature of the listing of categories. It was by memorizing classic citations, in order to later recite these Sanskrit phrases by heart and thus adorn and dignify anything they said with formulaic utterances, that Hindu doctors were trained to enumerate and combine categories with one another whenever they formulated a diagnosis, prognosis, or prescription in the course of medical consultations.

Take for example what is taught about cancer in Ayurvedic medicine. In the fascinating exposition of an Ayurvedic theory of cancer propounded by her guru Mahadeva Iyer in 1975 in southern Tamilnadu, Margaret Trawick (1991: 123) noted the fact that cancer receives scant attention in the texts, while modern Indian doctors devote considerable thought to it, at least in part, she suggested, because the Western biomedical description of this disease happens to fit very well the Ayurvedic paradigm of all diseases. Doctors say that *kapha* or phlegm is responsible for the growth of tumors. What is the rationale behind the image of phlegm? All diseases are cancers of some sorts as far as disease in general is a condition rather than the consequence of an invasion. The essential point in the Ayurvedic theory of cancer is that the abnormal growth of a tumor is not due to the presence of an invading agent but to a vitiated condition linked to birth itself. Cancer is a consequence of individuation and of the pollution or marking process inherent to any embodied being born in this world. On the plane of images, one might say that *vāta* is responsible for the faulty division of cells and *kapha* for their growth; this imagery of wind and phlegm is somewhat obscure. But Marriott's felicitous analytic language transposes the humoral theory into a tridimensional grid according to which cancer results from a combination of marking (pollution and tumescence), mixing (invasion), and unmatching (division and disorder). The dimension symbolized by *kapha* is that of marking, or pollution in a sheer physiological sense. As noted by Edwin Gerow in a precious vindication of Marriott's enterprise (2000: 415), the desacralization of the concept of pollution is made evident by calling it "marking." Disease is the normal state of the human body; health and even life itself are only maintained by medical attention. The living body is never without disease and embodiment in itself is a vitiated condition, because it is an assemblage of humors that are naturally at variance and contending with one another. This is a medical consequence of the Hindu and Buddhist philosophical doctrine according to which everything is pain and everybody is in pain at any given time.

Mahadeva Iyer's teachings and his demeanor in clinical practice illuminate two particular points. I shall first consider his views on cancer, which illustrated the dividuality of living beings. Then, to complete my presentation of an alternative ideology of health and disease, which clearly is not a simple matter of resistance to the dominant paradigm of biomedicine but is genuinely generated by a different philosophy, I shall later, following Trawick (1987), recall the ways this dedicated Ayurvedic practitioner expressed friendliness in his relating to patients, according to a principle of medical ethics which is just a corollary of the conception of dividual personhood. Let us summarize first what he said of cancer.

Cancer was illustrative of the demonic quality of life. Cancerous tumors seemed almost to take on a life of their own, eluding the would-be healer by taking numerous forms throughout the body, being suppressed here only to turn up again there. This was in consonance with the concept of a dividual person comprised of many beings with many different wills. Mahadeva Iyer borrowed from the Sanskrit texts metaphors and figures of speech like personification to refer to substances, processes, and organs in the body as if these substances, processes, and organs had wills and feelings of their own—the humors or the heart, for instance, could be angry or arrogant or hungry or tired or calm and happy. They were demons who should be worshipped lest they go astray, and cancerous tumors were examples of such internal components of the body ranging out of control. Pathology in Mahadeva Iyer's understanding did not follow an all-or-nothing logic; there did not exist any invasion, infection, or contagion process that could be stopped once and for all, nor any external invader that could be eradicated. He said that cancer might begin as an injury on the edge of some organ, and that the injury itself would become an organ and would grow, producing particles of pollution that would spread throughout the bloodstream (Trawick

1991: 125). There was a continuum and a vicious circle between injury and organ leading to a conflation of the two. A given injury did not heal, but rather grew, and in many forms joined with the flesh; a given wound every day grew bigger like a separate organ. Needless to say, the Aristotelian distinction between tissues and organs does not hold here. The difference between an injury and an organ was only a matter of proportion, an injured tissue evolving into a vitiated organ whenever things got out of order. In the same line of thought, Marriott (1990: 8) noted that all-or-nothing measures of an item's total presence or absence will rarely apply in traditional knowledge in India; all items of interest to the scholar—substances, processes, and components in a given organism—are variables. Each element and humor is said to be more or less strongly present everywhere at any time, just as disease, present at all times, is the natural condition of a living being, and health the elusive achievement of medical art. The very same processes and substances that are necessary for life are also responsible for illness and death. Boundaries are blurred between health and disease, between medicines and poisons, and between life and death, because—I am carefully choosing my words—this world is essentially dividual (or mixed), unbalanced (or marked), and chaotic (or unmatched).

The terminology used here to describe the fuzzy and demonic quality of substances and processes as they are described in traditional Indian medicine is modeled upon a set of anti-equivalence relations that were formulated by Marriott in a later phase of his work (Marriott 1990: 17; Gerow 2000: 419ff.). I shall omit the details and further references to the underlying mathematical model and concentrate on his main principle. The principle according to which all items taken into account in a diagnosis are variables already is an anti-equivalence relation. It means that all items are context-sensitive, that all relations among these items are necessarily particular, and that there is no transitivity nor consistency among these items. In Marriott's analytic language, the whole is "chaotic," "unmatched," and logically speaking "not transitive." Marriott's thesis that the many triads that prevail in various Hindu learned traditions constitute the universe as a set of anti-equivalence relations takes its full meaning when we apply it to the three humors of Ayurvedic medicine. *Pitta* symbolizes nonreflexive relations following which bodies and persons are mixed or dividual. *Kapha* symbolizes nonsymmetrical relations within the framework of which any set of given items is hierarchical or marked. *Vāta* symbolizes nontransitive relations which constitute any given universe as chaotic or unmatched. The matrix of cancer, in this alternative ideology of health and disease, is a set of physiological processes that are essentially nontransitive or unmatched (division of cells living a life of their own), and nonsymmetrical or marking (inordinate and demonic growth of tumors).

Now let us shift from the medical doctrine to the performance of medicine. Mahadeva Iyer's mode of discourse, the words he used, the tone of voice, and the body language differed with each audience. Always, in his discussions with those who visited him for treatment, he gave reasons for his diagnoses and the therapies he prescribed in a language of commitment and persuasion. He would seek a point of commonality between himself and each person he spoke with. He would invoke a common origin or a shared experience with his patients; he would extol agriculture for example whenever the patient happened to be a farmer—he himself owned about twenty acres of good paddy land and a dozen milk cows—or he would play on commonalities between professions, when the patient was a professional, and discuss the principles that medicine and art share. Trawick (1987: 1038) gives a juicy example of a play on words creating a sense of complicity with one of Iyer's patients who was a sculptor; he asked the sculptor to make for him a *śivaliṅgam* out of the poisonous/medicinal mineral cinnabar, the Sanskrit and Malayalam name of which is *jātiliṅgam,* thus suggesting that they were both experts on *liṅgam*! Establishing a connivance with all visitors might wrongly pass for a hypocritical sugarcoating of therapy, but this habit of seeking a point of commonality with each patient was essential to the process of diagnosis as well as to the choice of treatment. Even if the visitor was accompanied by family or friends, the doctor's communicative efforts were concentrated almost exclusively upon the individual patient. This seems to contradict the common scene described earlier in which the doctor, bypassing the patient, addresses his remarks to those in authority in the family or community. Actually, Mahadeva Iyer's intention was to address himself to community values and to the bond of nature existing between him and them. This idea of the existence of a bond of nature underlies humoralism, which in turn underlies the performance of medicine. This idea of a commonality among all creatures is just a corollary

111

of the conception of dividual personhood. The doctor's attitude was just expressing friendliness in the strict sense of the word and as a fundamental principle of medical ethics.

As it is taught in a quite explicit stanza of the *Carakasaṃhitā*, Sūtra 9.26, "Friendliness (*maitrī*) [toward all living beings], compassion (*kāruṇya*) for his patients, dedication (*prīti*) when [the disease is] curable, detachment (*upekṣaṇa*) towards living beings who are at the point of death: these are the physician's four rules of conduct." Cakrapāṇidatta glosses and comments the four key words as follows: "Which are the frames of mind (*buddhyāḥ*) that should be entertained by the physician, this is what the teacher explains in the stanza that reads '*maitrī* etc.' *Maitrī*: see the gloss at *Carakasaṃhitā*, Sūtra 8.29 [quoted below]. 'Patients': those who present with a complaint. *Kāruṇya*: one's desire to put an end to other people's suffering. 'Curable': when the physician is capable of curing the patient. Towards someone at the point of death, one should exercise detachment, abstaining from giving him medicines, for instance, lest it would destroy the [dying person's] *yaśas* [glory, dignity]." This is a quartet of Hindu categories teaching four rules of conduct and frames of mind to be adopted by the Ayurvedic physician according to circumstances. Dedication when the disease is curable and detachment toward a terminal patient are mere subdivisions of the category of compassion. Maintaining a compassionate demeanor toward one's own patients is a principle of medical ethics dictating two different rules of conduct depending on the physician's prognosis. One rule is to engage the disease when it is curable; another rule is to abstain from heroic measures that would unduly prolong the agony when the patient is dying. The Sanskrit texts thus formulate the right for all patients to die with dignity, and more exactly, the right for a terminally ill to preserve one's Glory (*yaśas*), that is all values that will be transmitted to later rebirths. The most important value, however, is that of friendliness (*maitrī*).

Friendliness, in this particular context, is the acknowledgment of a bond of nature among all living beings. To quote Cakrapāṇidatta's gloss at *Carakasaṃhitā*, Sūtra 8.29: *maitrī sarvabhūteṣv ātmanīvāpratikūlā pravṛttiḥ*, "Friendliness is an unrestricted kindness to all creatures as to oneself." I would like to suggest that this ethical principle was exactly what inspired Mahadeva Iyer with regard to his attitude and efforts to connect patients not only or necessarily with himself, but with other patients or loved ones that he had cared for in the past. Therefore his demeanor was built upon his experiences with persons and the conviction that this world was made up of fragmented selves sharing parts of themselves with one another because there was no strict line of demarcation between persons and things. "From the blade of grass to Brahmā," as the Sanskrit phrase goes, there seemed to be a continuum along which tissues, organs, and bodies could alternatively be characterized as individuated persons or things and parts of one another.

Are such conceptions specific to India? One cannot say. The idea of a commonality between persons and things is not unknown in the West, where it has been discussed since at least the eighteenth century. Ethical debates on the eighteenth-century distinction between the "instrumental" value of a thing understood as a spare part of something else and the "intrinsic" value of a thing personified as a self-contained organism have been of considerable importance. The former is the value of things as means to further some other ends, whereas the latter is the value of things as ends in themselves regardless of whether they are also useful as means to other ends. For example, a certain wild plant may have instrumental value because it provides the ingredients for some medicine. But if the plant also has some value in itself independently of its prospects for furthering some other ends such as human health, then the plant also has an intrinsic value that generates a moral duty on the part of moral agents to protect it or at least refrain from damaging it. This is why contemporary jurists, in the context of ecological activism, have argued that herbs and trees did "have standing" and could be defended by lawyers in court as if they were persons. This distinction between the instrumental value of a thing and the intrinsic value of a person's experience is an anthropocentric idea based on the concept of nature alternatively defined in the West as fit for possession—*humans mastering and possessing Nature* (Descartes)—and entitled to respect—*Nature is so fragile*. A similar conflation of things and values is to be found in the Indian concept of *artha*. Just as our concept of nature, however, is not readily transferable to Asian worldviews, reciprocally, the Sanskrit word *artha* is not satisfactorily construed in terms of "things" and "values," although "thing" and "value" are both perfectly valid translations of Sanskrit *artha*. In the learned traditions of Hindu and Buddhist philosophy as well as in local knowledge in India, our relationship to herbs and trees has never been experienced as purely objectival nor aesthetic nor instrumental. Herbs and trees have sometimes if not quite often been thought of as dividual persons just like parts of the human body. Our relationship to herbs and trees and other living beings has been experienced as foundational of the great chain of *saṃsāra*, the wheel of rebirths, and it has been construed as "iconic," if I may borrow this word from semiotics, meaning that we share our own substance and personality with them. This is the philosophical basis of the Hindu concept of dividual persons.

Was not it already said in the *Chāndogya Upaniṣad* 6.11 when Āruṇi shows his son Śvetaketu a tall tree that is being pruned, trimmed, and mutilated by all means, but still grows constantly new suckers? Even as you make a gash in its root or its trunk, "pervaded by the living (*jīva*) self (*ātman*)," it remains happy, greedily sucking the saps from the soil. Although it usually means "living being," the word *jīva* points here to what makes the tree living, the life principle in it, an essence that does not receive life from external causes but pursues life from its own liveliness. The division of matter and life is not always explicitly made or even admitted in the various philosophical schools of India. In the *Chāndogya* version of an environmental ethics that is holistic and foundational, all living creatures—from gods through twigs and herbs—are endowed with *karma*. In the same line of thought, Uddyotakara's *Nyāyavārttika* 4.1.47 teaches that if somebody waters a tree, the success of his action, that is, the process of fertilization and growth, may be influenced by the *karma* of the person who at a later time will eat the fruits of the tree. Life is a bond that ties together all living beings along the great chain of living beings that unwinds over the *saṃsāra*. What sets matter apart from life is the absence of *karma* causality. Conversely, the implication of the doctrine of *saṃsāra* seems to be that there is no life without *karma*, that life and *saṃsāra*, the two realms of biology and soteriology, are exactly coextensive.

Disease Inherent to Individuation

Indian views on individuation were the point of departure of this inquiry into situations in which medical sciences and local knowledge intersect to produce alternative ideologies of health and disease. This chapter is based on the presupposition that the set of anti-equivalence relations underlying Indian views on individuation were worth studying for themselves. My ambition was to pursue the analysis beyond the point at which TCAM and specifically "traditional medicine" are simply "resisting," that is merely reactive to, the advent of biomedicine and medical individualism. Disease, according to South Asian classical teachings, is ingrained in the nature of a born being because of individuation; disease is a mixed condition produced by the superimposition of different levels of reality in the patient's body. I have tried to demonstrate that a dead corpse and the skin of an individual body only seem to delineate clear-cut boundaries between life and death and between the self and the other as long as the transitory lived world in which we were born dissimulates its nonreflexive, nonsymmetrical, and nontransitive structure.

A second presupposition was that no medical condition could be assessed or even described without language. We focused our attention on language and verbal performance in medical consultations. Utterances and statements, in the course of medical encounters between patients and healers, were contextualized from the angle of addressivity. It is through speech events and in the course of what is called in Sanskrit *vyavahāra,* "the conversation, interactions with others," that we participate in the reality of those we differentiate ourselves from, as when a clinician is faced with a patient. Diagnoses, prognoses, and prescriptions are matters for discourse and dialogue, and medical practice has traditionally taken the form of a conversation, although the advent of sophisticated investigation technologies relegated language to a position of secondary importance.

In the opinion of a modern clinician quoted above—"that word 'God willing' gives them as easy way out"—discourse and dialogue in traditional and alternative medicine tend to be justificatory. I would like to strongly deny such an assertion and I hope this chapter has shown that language in the performance of learned traditional medicine, far from being used as a set of hypocritical and rhetorical devices to please the patient and justify potential failures, provided doctors with the necessary keys of interpretation. Three levels of reality— therefore three causalities—have been defined in classical Ayurveda, namely: *yukti* (human reasoning and natural conjunctions), *sattva* (willpower or human agency), and *daiva* (the wheel of rebirths). The boundaries separating each one from the others in our usual understanding are blurred, yielding confusion first between humans and nature (meaning other living beings like herbs and trees), second between the physical and the mental, and last but not least between life and death. The fact that the demarcation line between life and death is blurred plays an essential role in some special areas of medicine, like infertility medicine or organ transplants. What yields uncertainty between therapeutic success and failure eventually is not the conflation of the rational with the metaphysical, as was asserted by the sociologists quoted in the beginning of this chapter, but the ambiguity inscribed in life itself and the superimposition of different levels of reality in one and the same living body.

Notes

1. A further 5 percent of respondents were interviewed with an accompanying family member.
2. Successful cases are fully documented in the TKDL archives.
3. The modern habit of recording medical case histories in English seems to have appeared in Ayurvedic hospitals and nursing homes from the 1960s on, as far as I can tell.
4. http://www.vasudevaayurvedics.com/stroke.htm. Accessed 28 May 2010.

References

Bharadwaj, Aditya. 2003. "Why Adoption Is Not an Option in India: The Visibility of Infertility, the Secrecy of Donor Insemination, and Other Cultural Complexities." *Social Science and Medicine* 56: 1867–1880.

———. 2006. "Sacred Conceptions: Clinical Theodicies, Uncertain Science, and Technologies of Procreation in India." *Culture, Medicine and Psychiatry* 30: 451–465.

———. 2008. "Biosocialities and Biocrossings: Encounters with Assisted Conception and Embryonic Stem Cells in India." In *Biosocialities, Genetics and the Social Sciences: Making Biologies and Identities,* ed. Sahra Gibbon and Carlos Novas. Abingdon and New York: Routledge, 98–116.

Broom, Alex, Assa Doron, and Philip Tovey. 2009. "The Inequalities of Medical Pluralism: Hierarchies of Health, the Politics of Tradition and the Economies of Care in Indian Oncology." *Social Science & Medicine* 69: 698–706.

Gerow, Edwin. 2000. "India as a Philosophical Problem: McKim Marriott and the Comparative Enterprise." *Journal of the American Oriental Society* 120(3) (July–September): 410–429.

Marriott, McKim. 1990. "Constructing an Indian Ethnosociology." In *India Through Hindu Categories,* ed. McKim Marriott. New Delhi: Sage Publications, 1–39.

Tovey, Philip, and Alex Broom. 2007. "Oncologists' and Specialist Cancer Nurses' Approaches to Complementary and Alternative Medicine and their Impact on Patient Action." *Social Science & Medicine* 64: 2550–2564.

Trawick, Margaret. 1987. "The Ayurvedic Physician as Scientist." *Social Science and Medicine* 24(12): 1031–1050.

———.1991. "An Ayurvedic Theory of Cancer." *Medical Anthropology* 13: 121–136. Reprinted 1992 in *Anthropological Approaches to the Study of Ethnomedicine,* ed. Mark Nichter. Yverdon: Gordon and Breach, 207–222.

Chapter Four
My *Vaidya* and
My Gynecologist
Agency, Authority, and
Risk in Quest of a Child

Harish Naraindas

The Institution of Hospitalized Birthing

For most urban women worldwide, the default mode for a birthing experience is a hospital. In the Euro-American world, birth in a hospital is nearly universal, and only about 3 to 4 percent of births occur outside its portals in two of its largest economies, namely, the United States and Germany.[1] In urban India, especially in its large metropolises, the numbers are even higher, with cities like Madras (now Chennai) registering an impressive 99 percent of institutional deliveries, either through sub-health centers, primary care centers, district hospitals, or tertiary hospitals (Padmanabhan 2008).[2] The hospital is the sine qua non of a "modern" birthing experience and "birthing women who resist the medicalization of pregnancy and childbirth are considered a risk to their unborn baby and in many situations coerced into complying with medical recommendations for the sake of their baby" (MacKinnon and McIntyre 2006: 59).

The notion of risk, which is fundamental in modern medicine, especially post World War II,[3] seems particularly pronounced in the case of pregnancy, indeed doubly so as the mother and her behavior may be construed as being "risky" for the "unborn child."[4] While this may be especially the case in a society as litigious as the United States, we will see the palpable presence of "risk" in this chapter and how it haunts the narrative of the main protagonist in India at every turn.[5] Some have argued that this contemporary framing of risk has led to a set of hospital protocols that are nothing but *rituals,* as there is little or no evidence to support these practices (MacKinnon and McIntyre 2006: 59). Hence, hospital births with their associated *rituals* of the lithotomic position, the fetal monitor, the epidural, the episiotomy, etc. (Davis-Floyd 1990),[6] along with perhaps childhood vaccinations, are best seen as rites of passage through which "modern subjects" are fashioned and are either near universal or sought to be made near universal by modernizing states. Therefore it comes as no surprise that in my eight years of teaching a course on the anthropology of childbirth and pregnancy on three continents, successive batches of students look puzzled when I ask them in an opening gambit as to where they (or their prospective wives/partners) intend to give birth. For almost all of them, including young women who may see themselves as feminists, it is, till that moment of reckoning, taken for granted that their prospective birthing experience either for themselves or their future partners would be in a hospital. A few women, and almost exclusively women, are unsure; and even fewer (not more than ten out of about 200 students in the eight years) say rather hesitantly that they do not wish to give birth in a hospital, or state unambiguously that they prefer to have it at home or in a free-standing birth center, attended by midwives rather than doctors (this statement coming only from students in the United States and Germany). One of my students did indeed give birth in such a center, and another wanted to have one in the sea with dolphins for company (both these in Germany).[7] In a few more cases women intended to have a home birth but were either redeemed or fell prey to a hospital birth as first a "disease," and then the *discipline* called obstetrics, an *institution* called the hospital, and a professional *practice* called gynecology, either saved or ambushed them.

Of these four categories—disease, discipline, institution, and practice—the most insidious may well be the category called "disease" because it is very difficult for most modern subjects to imagine multiple nosologies, even while they may imagine other institutions (such as free-standing birth centers), other professions (such as midwives) and other disciplines, or systems (such as homeopathy, phytotherapy, or anthroposophy). By and large in the West these other systems, professions, and institutions subscribe to virtually the same

119

nosology, perhaps with certain cardinal differences in inflection and at times radical differences in treatment; or, more fundamentally but increasingly rarely, what is understood as laryngitis (for example) in one system (biomedicine) may not be understood in quite the same way in Homeopathy. In India, however (and perhaps elsewhere too), multiple nosologies are *nominally* possible. It is this nominal possibility that is in part responsible for the narrative to follow and has led me to christen the quandary it leads to as *nosopolitics*.[8] This is due, in part, to the existence of other state-sanctioned systems of medicine and to the widespread existence of other "marginalized systems" without state backing.[9] These other systems (like Ayurveda), or the ones described by several of the authors in this volume, unlike in the West, often have fully elaborated alternative nosologies,[10] although in the last 100 years or so, the state sanctioned ones like Ayurveda, Unani, and Siddha have been mangled if not altogether recast and creolized (Naraindas 2014) by an asymmetrical conversation with allopathy, resulting in the reshaping of pedagogy and the production of handbooks where Ayurvedic therapies are now offered for a biomedical nosology (Naraindas 2006).

In what follows I recount the story of a middle-class woman in urban India who sought to avoid a hospital birth by turning to Ayurveda. I intend to show, through a retrospective narrative of her experience, what this entailed and how she equivocated and struggled to negotiate her career as a patient or prospective mother between competing forms of authority and expertise. In fact, one of the fulcrums around which this chapter revolves is the *experiential consequence* of attempting to negotiate the potential minefield created by such competing forms of expertise. At the end of this recounting, I also hope to interrogate and partially call into question some of the models and theories that have been deployed in medical anthropology to understand the dynamics of what is called "health-seeking behavior."

Before I do so, I offer a schematic and comparative picture of India, the United States, and Germany with respect to hospital birthing and its alternatives, including what I have called postmodern forms of birthing, in order to better understand where things stand in India vis-à-vis the Euro-American world, which, in global public health discourse as well as in the discourse of development, invariably functions as both norm and critique of the Third World.

Hence, in the following two sections I move between East and West in an attempt to compare and reciprocally clarify the issue. I must also state before I proceed that this single retrospective narrative is based on an ethnographic study of an Ayurvedic practitioner in South India based on six months of continuous participant observation in her clinic, and subsequent visits lasting from a few days to a few weeks over the course of two years. I spoke to about 500 patients as part of my study, observed their therapy and interaction with the practitioner, and met several of them at home and elsewhere. I interviewed some of them (including Sangita, the main protagonist below) several times both in and outside the clinic in an attempt to understand their therapeutic/childbirth quest. This chapter is also based on fieldwork in the United States (and some in Germany and the U.K.), where the main thrust was on "natural/home births," as part of which I spoke with women, spouses/partners, mothers, prospective mothers, nurses, nurse-midwives, lay midwives, *doulas,* obstetricians, pediatricians, pathologists, morticians, undertakers, priests, and pastors. In the United States, as in India, my initial six months of fieldwork in and around a very large teaching hospital were followed by several visits over subsequent years, and included stints in the university women's resource center, an abortion clinic, local churches, and in the company of "pro-life" activists belonging to an evangelical organization and classes on Calvin in a local church conducted by a university professor and Pulitzer Prize winner. Hence, this single narrative is embedded in a multisited and comparative fabric, in an attempt to show that "local" narratives are both singular and at the same time part of larger "circulating" global forms (Appadurai 2010).

Of Hospital and Home Births in the United States and India

Unlike in North America or Europe, with their spectrum of home-birth advocates, be they hippies, midwives, the far right, feminists, the Amish, or anthropologists, there are almost no home-birth advocates in India; and virtually no published cases of *intended* home births, with the lone exception of Manju Kapur, the Delhi-based novelist and professor of English literature at the University of Delhi, who gave birth to her fourth child virtually unattended in her house near Khan Market in central Delhi (Kapur 2006). Home births in India are either of rural provenance (65 percent in rural India), or occur among the urban poor (Haq 2008). This is partly because the educated *urban* middle class has little or no access to lay midwives, as is the case in the United States,[11] nor to "certified nurse midwives" in the hospital, whom they may see independently of the doctor for their entire course of pregnancy, which is by now de rigueur in the United States. Such professions hardly exist in urban India, while in rural India "midwives," *dais,* and trained birth attendants (TBAs)[12] are ubiquitous and are assiduously promoted by the state in an effort to persuade rural women to deliver their children in a medical institution under these forms of *expert paramedical* supervision. In urban India, and particularly for middle-class women, there is only the faintest glimmer of the possibility of a non-hospital-based delivery. This has partly to do with the country's institutional setup and partly with the fact that in the minds of educated middle-class women, "home delivery" is coeval with all that is rural, backward, and therefore risky.

Images of danger and risk are deliberately underlined by the modernizing Indian state, as it continues to promote institutionalized birthing for the residual rural majority and the poor urban minority as *the solution* to the high rate of infant and maternal mortality.[13] In fact the hospital delivery, with its associated rituals of the episiotomy and the caesarean, has become so successful in India that while the WHO mandates a 10 percent rate for episiotomies, it is virtually 100 percent in private hospitals in (some parts of) the country and 98 percent in tertiary postgraduate teaching hospitals run by the state (Selvaraj et al. 2007);[14] and while caesareans vary between 7 to 25 percent in the Euro-American world,[15] the rate might be as high as 47 percent or more in private hospitals in a city like Chennai (Sreevidya and Sathiyasekaran 2003). In Germany, according to the president of the German midwives association, whom I interviewed in 2010, although on average only every third birth is a caesarean, there are certain well-known hospitals (she mentioned one in Cologne), where births can be virtually 100 percent C-sections. This also seems to be the case, according to some of my informants, in certain hospitals in South Madras, where my story is set. While I cannot guarantee the accuracy of either of these figures, they are best read as an index of institutions across the world that are well known for very high C-section rates, and may well be the result of what are called elective caesareans chosen by the well-to-do, which in the Anglo-Saxon context is best summed up by the adage "too posh to push," made popular by the English press when the Spice Girl Posh chose an elective caesarean in March 1999. The current caesarean rates in Germany and the United States may be testimony to the fact that this adage not only reflects a widespread attitude but also translates into high caesarean rates in the Euro-American world, while in the Third World, the caesarean, like the episiotomy, is often even more pronounced. What is evident from these figures is that state promotion of institutional birthing, along with educational socialization into a scientific worldview, has become so ubiquitous that it outlives all political regimes.[16]

In India this persistence is compounded by the fact that hospital deliveries introduce new twists in the prestation and counterprestation economy that marks marriage and kinship in South Asia where, for many if not most communities and regions, the woman goes to the natal house for her delivery, especially of the first child. The cost and care of this first birth is usually borne by the natal household, and it is expected that this will be done, like many of the rituals that mark the nine months of pregnancy,[17] with care and concern if not with pomp and show. The hospital as a site partly exacerbates and partly transforms the trajectory of a contemporary pregnancy, and especially an urban middle-class pregnancy. It often leads women, households, and kin networks to embrace the C-section for reasons of status, apart from its purported claim of being safe and painless.[18] In this status economy, the caesarean may resituate the middle-class South Asian woman away from the axis of purity and pollution and a vaginal birth (though this is moot), into a medical setting and a surgical birth, with interesting subplots and fallouts.

Apart from physician-driven and institutionally driven reasons for C-sections (namely, the well-known nine-to-five and Monday-to-Friday C-section births), these subplots may derive from patients' demand, which was also the third most common reason for an elective caesarean section in the U.K. in 1992 (Atiba et al. 1993). While this demand is usually attributed to the need to avoid labor pain, another common reason seems to stem from the belief that a vaginal delivery would spoil a woman's future sexual performance and her husband's pleasure (Mello e Souza 1994). In addition to these reasons, in India, as Kabra et al. (1994) have pointed out, there is the astrological calendar and the need for births to occur at a predetermined auspicious time.[19] The episiotomy, too, like the C-section, has a dubious "sexual history," apart from all the purportedly medical reasons made in its favor, namely, that the straight surgical incision, as opposed to the unseemly natural tear, could be neatly stitched (aesthetics), and "stitched tight" for a good "family life." In other words, if one is to have a vaginal delivery instead of a C-section, the episiotomy allegedly helps ensure pleasure. In fact, the wife of one of my informants in the United States not only gave birth in a hospital despite her best intentions, but was also, to her utter dismay, subjected to an episiotomy. My informant reports that as he was stitching her up, the obstetrician turned to him and said, "Dick, this extra one is for you."

The end result of these plots and subplots is that a caesarean often acquires snob value,[20] best exemplified by the adage "too posh to push"; and quite like the price range of pacemakers (from 50,000 to 500,000 rupees), or varieties of tooth fillings (porcelain, silver, or gold), it enters into a hierarchical structure of the preferred way of giving birth, compounded by the prestige of the hospital, its décor, its zip-code, the doctor, her degrees, and so forth. In India, this *prestige economy* feeds into the garrulous postbirth chatter of the endless stream of visitors of the near and extended kin who come visiting at the hospital. But the other side of this phenomenal success, or what in the anthropological literature is called the "medicalization of birthing," is that at least some of these same middle-class Indian women are now aware of perceived problems with caesarean deliveries, which is so ubiquitous that among certain social classes it is virtually impossible to meet a woman in an Indian metropolis who has *not* had one.

But the critique of the caesarean is largely couched in terms of its political economy, where doctors and especially hospitals are seen as performing them for commercial gain.[21] This critique usually does not translate into looking for "alternatives," as it indeed does not for the 97 or 98 percent of German or American women who still give birth in the hospital.[22] However, for these German and American women this has resulted in what could be called the "natural birth movement," where a growing number of prospective mothers, in the last thirty years or so, are seen by certified nurse-midwives (CNMs) rather than doctors and delivered by these CNMs "naturally," that is, without an episiotomy, let alone a caesarean—and if possible with no epidurals (spinal anesthesia) or an amniotomy, resulting in a "natural" and often prolonged labor.[23] But this "natural birth" resurgence is largely within the confines of the hospital, which see the alternative birthing centers, and the lay midwifery movement (in the United States), as potential competitors that they have to counter to retain their clientele.

This became evident to me at the end of a year (2003–2004) of fieldwork at one of the largest teaching hospitals in the United States and is based on interviews with nurse-midwives, lay midwives (illegal in this particular state), women who had given birth in the new birthing center at the hospital, others who had given birth at home, their husbands/partners, and *doulas*. I twice attended day-long birthing classes, where we were taken on a tour of the "new" birthing room, where the birthing instructor put one of the male partners on the table and used him as a live birthing model to simulate the possible trajectories that the birthing woman may go through on "birthing day." I also invited two nurse-midwives to address my students, during which the senior nurse-midwife (with forty years of experience) quite clearly told the class that "we'll do what it takes to keep the competition out; and if it means putting in a Jacuzzi so that they can have an underwater birth massaged by water jets, then so be it." In fact, a bathtub, if not a Jacuzzi, is by now de rigueur in many if not most hospitals.[24] One presumes this is increasingly the case with the new birthing table, which was a technological marvel that twisted, turned, and decomposed, thus allowing the birthing woman to assume a variety of positions rather than being merely supine and hence "disempowered"—apparently without "disempowering" the nurse-midwife or the obstetrician, who could still "stand up" (rather than squat) and "catch the baby."[25] It is thus evident that birthing, at least at this historical juncture, is an ongoing and evolving conversation, if not an agon, between the hospital and its critics.

In India in 2001–2003, when I conducted the fieldwork on which this chapter is based, there was no "natural birth" *movement* either in or out of the hospital, though "natural birthing" within the confines of the hospital has now emerged. However, what was available to a small class of well-informed women was the critique of hospital births, which they saw as enormously commercialized and hence disempowering, since financial profit, rather than the health of the woman, was seen to be at the center of the whole business, leading some of them to look for alternatives.

But turning toward an alternative, as I will presently show, is fraught with risk; and attempts to circumvent that which is general and common invites trouble, since the general and the common are external and constraining and hence, as Durkheim (1982) would say, "social facts." I intend to show through a retrospective narrative of one young woman's experience what an attempted breach of *social facts* may entail and, through it, to partially call into question some of the theories that have been deployed in medical anthropology to understand the dynamics of what is often called the "doctor–patient interaction," a subcategory of "health-seeking behavior." Part of my claim in this chapter is that much available writing in the medical humanities is situated at best between the "culture" of patients and the "science" of doctors with their disciplines, professions, and institutions; and as a homologue of the same, between what is called disease (the provenance of doctors) and illness (the provenance of patients) (Mol 2002). I suggest that what we witness instead in this young woman's retrospective narrative are (at least) two competing but asymmetrical modes of expert authority and the attempt to exercise agency in their shadow, leading to a wager on the part of the patient against the likelihood of death, deformity, and guilt, since the patient/prospective mother, buffeted while negotiating a moral, medical, and economic minefield, can rely neither on a single form of embodied authority, nor on a vade mecum that will *go with her* in her travails.

Ayurveda and the Possibility of Postmodern Birthing

In the American context, we now have a postmodern birthing room, if not a hospital, which is aware of the growing competition from standalone birthing centers, or alternative birthing centers (ABCs), and from the vibrant community of lay midwives. It is clear that the hospital has over the years attempted to counter and "absorb" this critical community within its precincts, in terms of both personnel (by creating a new class of professionals called certified nurse-midwives or CNMs), and architecture (by refurbishing the birthing room and the birthing table and introducing, among other things, a bathtub/Jacuzzi). In this new setting, the male partner occupies pride of place at the head of the birthing woman, and he is there not by chance or by default but is present after being schooled elaborately through cohort birthing classes into a new etiquette of "cobirthing" and "being there" for the woman. He, along with the latest lay professional, the *doula*,[26] is advocate, "midwife," and mediation between the birthing woman and the certified nurse-midwife and hospital staff, and is there to ensure that the "twenty-point" program of natural birth that his partner has drawn up (often in consultation with him and her *doula*) is adhered to.

In Japan, *postmodern birthing,* if one can call it that, has also taken the form of *clinics* run by mid-wives who have had formal training in modern hospitals—supplemented by other kinds of traditional techniques learnt from a generation of midwives before hospital delivery became the norm. These postmodern clinics, rather than concentrating on the "delivery as cardinal event," register and run the women through her entire pregnancy and provide both antenatal and postpartum care, quite like lay midwives in the United States, or in other parts of the world where the hospital has not yet penetrated—with a good example being the case of the midwife Dona in the Yucatan described by Jordan (Jordan 1983). While some of these women seem to have supplemented their training and experience with "premodern" techniques, they have come to be connected (by means of an umbilical cord?) to the hospital, with an obstetrician available in case of "complications."

The birthing house (*Geburtshaus*) in Germany and elsewhere in Europe is a variation of this, where, although trained midwives are the mainstay, there is sometimes a doctor on the premises or on call, or the birth house is tied to a hospital for use in the case of an emergency.[27] In Germany such birth houses are, in fact, a parallel resource to the hospital and may be paid for by "socialized compulsory insurance," though not as easily or as fully as hospital births. Hence their form, expertise and personnel requirements are partly determined by protocols laid down by health insurance and often resemble to a greater or lesser extent protocols in the hospital, though with seemingly small (and at times significant) differences that to discerning women may have enormous consequences both in terms of outcome and the experience of birthing.[28] In the U.K., although the birth may be at home, a nurse-midwife from the hospital attends it and treats the patient and the event as a kind of hospital outreach program, and hence appears with all the medical paraphernalia that may be necessary for the birth.[29]

The glaring exception to this ubiquitous norm of the hospital birth in the Euro-American world seems to be the "Dutch way of birth," where in an otherwise high-tech biomedical environment, nearly one-third of all births occur at home. Dutch midwives attend 71 percent of all home births and 48 percent of all births, resulting in one of the lowest infant mortalities and lowest surgical interventions worldwide. This has led to two schools of Dutch obstetrics, one of which, deeply embarrassed by this anomaly, attempts to collect statistics to decry it. These research findings are published in the United States, where they "are deemed scientific," and not published in Holland where they are deemed "not scientific." The other school, which is proud of the Dutch way of birth, has its research findings in support of this mode published in Holland, where they are deemed scientific and not published in the United States, where they are not deemed scientific (De Vries et al. 2008)!

In India, none of these alternative, complementary, or postmodern institutional forms, with their graded structure from "natural birth" inside a high-tech hospital, to partially medicalized alternative birthing centers, or a community of lay midwives who reject obstetricians and hospitals, exist. Instead, I examine the case of a doctor (*vaidya*) formally trained (five and a half years) in one of the Indian systems of medicine, namely, Ayurveda, who guides the expectant mother through the entire period of pregnancy. I must further add that her clinic houses within its premises a yoga center, which is handled by her longtime associate and cofounder. The regimen of Ayurveda and yoga that the women are put through suggest interesting parallels to the various forms of natural and alternative birthing that we have alluded to. Practicing in South Madras with a large (but not solely) middle- and upper-class clientele she (read *they*, depending on the context), like the Japanese clinics, or the ABCs in the United States, seems to point to a future of *hybrid* births in India. A small but increasing number of women have put themselves under her care for the entire period of their pregnancy. However, since she does not deliver the children,[30] they are also simultaneously under the care of a gynecologist, who is the one who delivers the child in a hospital/private maternity clinic.

Unlike the well-networked postmodern clinics and midwives of Japan, or the *Geburthaus* in Germany, or even the Lay Midwives (LMs) in the United States where lay midwifery is legal, this *vaidya* consciously *contests* the "modern" in all its forms, thus positing her system as an alternative to the reigning orthodoxy.[31] Hence, as she often put it to me, the fact that she did not deliver children "is a personal limitation and not the limitation of my science";[32] and at least some of her clients would have been more than happy had she done so.[33]

We must also keep in mind another difference. Unlike professional midwives in the United States (either CNMs or LMs), or unlike even the gynecologist, the *vaidya* is, as an approximate category and to use the language of allopathic orthodoxy, a general physician. Here I use the second half of the description far more literally, insofar as she carries out no "surgery." This is largely if not wholly due to the way she has been trained, which again is almost wholly due to the fact that Ayurvedic surgery is largely a "dead" practice compared to its theoretical elaboration.[34] But insofar as she is a general physician she handles all kinds of cases, much like a homeopath. However, unlike an allopathic GP, she does not refer her patients to either a specialist or to a modern hospital but sees herself as effectively the last port of call. Since she is a "generalist," her female patients initially came to her for other ailments and, "having tasted the fruits," decided to put themselves under her care for their pregnancies. Because she did not deliver children in her clinic, patients were forced to run a dual course between two practitioners and two systems of medicine.

This dual course often resulted in clear conflicts, especially at times of crisis. I examine one such retrospective narrative (and weave other narratives into it) to indicate how the women negotiate this minefield. In this negotiation, terms like "syncretism" and "pluralism" (Leslie 1992), which are often used to characterize contemporary Ayurvedic practice in India, may not be very useful. Instead, this narrative offers us a commentary on lay and expert knowledge, notions of authority, agency, and decision making, and most importantly on the epistemic and ontological politics between two systems of medicine. It also invites us to reflect on the *politics* of childbirth as *idea*, *practice*, and *institution*, or as modes of thought and codes of conduct that constrain and channel the narrative when someone attempts to circumvent or sidestep it.

Choice and Risk: Alternative Paths and the Risk of Deformed Babies

Sangita is a web-page designer and multimedia expert whose father was completely cured of his severe diabetes by a *siddha vaidya* (a doctor of "Tamil medicine"). She too was treated by a *bogar*[35] for her irregular periods. Unable, after some time, to take the *bogar's* excruciatingly bitter and "nauseating" brew first thing in the morning, she approached Teresa (the Ayurvedic *vaidya*/doctor) in December 2001. Teresa treated her and after one cycle her periods stopped. Teresa told her that she was probably pregnant and asked her to return in March. Sangita meanwhile saw a gynecologist, was run through a test and declared pregnant. Although Sangita liked Teresa, she did not have a warm, personal relationship with her. She often described Teresa as a stern and slightly distant figure, unlike her gynecologist who seemed to have a wonderful bedside manner. "But it was one of the few moments that she was very happy when I announced the fact [her pregnancy] to her and she very warmly invited me to come see her soon. But she didn't realize that it was going to be, right from the beginning, a big fight."

Friends and family advised Sangita against experimenting with her life and with the new life of her baby. She, too, was acutely aware of the fact that she "had to be responsible and couldn't afford to be a guinea pig." Since the child was going to be the first grandchild on both sides of the family, there was enormous pressure to conform. Her father, who had earlier recounted his rather "miraculous" cure story to me, was a trenchant opponent and had accused her of experimenting with a quack,[36] while his own *siddha vaidya* (a Fellow of a Royal College of Surgeons (FRCS) from Edinburgh turned renegade) was a self-taught *vaidya* who lived on a farm, ran an orphanage, dispensed medicines with no "label," and lived entirely on tender coconut water and a small lump of clay once a day.

Her first shock came in the form of a friend and young mother asking her if she had been put on folic acid and when she said no she was told that her child was going to be born without a backbone. "Tell me, if you were pregnant, how would you react?" she asked me. I made it worse by telling her that I had had a long session with Vidya, another of Teresa's patients then into her eighth month of

130

pregnancy, and that Vidya had indeed had folic acid, convinced that her child would otherwise be born with spina bifida, or neural tube disorder, resulting, I said, in a "forked spine."

Sangita, on hearing this, immediately picked up her child, turned him over, and started intensely examining the base of his spine to see if it was forked. She began running her thumb and forefinger along its base: and slowly, as I watched, her fingers seem to unconsciously grow apart into a fork. When I left Sangita many hours later, this image stayed with me and I realized that this was a gesture she might well repeat in the days to come.

I must pause here for a moment and confess that I had to fight the urge to stroke the base of my own spine when I saw Sangita intensely stroking the base of her child's spine. I consoled myself by saying that I had not made it worse by telling her that Vidya had also, as part of her own panic, told me that the lack of folic acid could also lead to "babies without a brain." But "such babies," as I discovered later, usually die, while the fetuses with spinal disorders used to die but are now rescued and rehabilitated by (often repeated) surgery. I discovered this through a long and agonizing sit in at the pediatric department of "my" university teaching hospital in the United States, among a prospective "spina bifida mother," a special nurse for rehabilitation, and an assistant professor and clinician of pediatrics. One of the things the prospective mother wanted to know was whether the *rehabilitation* included the possibility of her possible future son being able to reproduce, have sex, and be able to find a viable partner, and quite how, if he was going to be born paralyzed from waist downward. While all this was answered (with the help of a large, stuffed, toy-child) in the affirmative with caveats, it appeared to me that "new technologies" made certain kinds of life "possible" and in the same breath brought in its wake amazing moral, economic, and psychological predicaments for persons/patients now presented with choices that would have been unthinkable without these technologies and their attendant social technologies for the differently able.[37] Apart from presenting patients with choice and risk as obverse sides of the same coin, what these medical and attendant social technologies seemed to do was make themselves a sine qua non for a childbirth experience. Any attempt to sidestep them was not merely fraught, presumably making the mother's behavior risky for the child, but it brought in its wake the possibility of life-long guilt, tellingly borne out by Sangita's anxious examination of the back of her perfectly healthy child.

Sangita had already been to Teresa in the past for her husband's asthma and had learned to respect her abilities. She had decided, even before conception, that she was going to put herself under her care and would have gladly not seen a gynecologist if Teresa had also undertaken to deliver the child. But the risk of having a "baby without a backbone" frightened her. When I asked Sangita how she had negotiated it, she said that she immediately had the folic acid for a day. She then proceeded to speak to her friend Sumitra, who had delivered her child under Teresa's care. Sumitra told her, said Sangita, to "blindly and wholly submit herself" to Teresa and had laughed the folic acid out of court by saying, "These are ridiculous norms probably laid down by the WHO, which presumes that all women in the third world are malnourished. And if this was true, all of us should have been spineless!"

Sumitra then reminded Sangita of a mutual friend of theirs, who had her first child at the age of forty-three entirely under Teresa's care, and how both mother and child were now doing fine. Sumitra had concluded by saying, "Quietly submit yourself to Teresa and make sure you start your yoga in the fourth month." This conversation reassured Sangita and, as she put it, "for someone at forty-three to do that was a leap of faith. But the first thing I did was to examine the child when it was born to see if it had ten fingers and ten toes. There is an enormous guilt attached to giving birth to deformed babies."

I presumed that this was the kind of fear and guilt that had not allowed Vidya to take any "risks" with the folic acid, irrespective of her otherwise dogged commitment to the dietary regimen prescribed by Teresa.

Teresa's Pregnancy Regimen

The regimen consisted of a diet of milk and rice (or wheat porridge) at least twice a day and, if possible, for all three meals. Lentils and pulses were largely proscribed as they increased *vāta*, and nothing cold in temperature, either by way of food or drink, as it also increased *vāta*. She was also advised to have buttermilk instead of yogurt, but never to have it as part of a meal that consisted of milk.

Nothing sour was to be consumed, which meant virtually no fruit (as most fruits are sour or have a sour aftertaste), with pomegranate as a cardinal exception, which in fact was positively recommended. Only a few of the large range of vegetables, and nothing that grew underground as it increased *vāta,* and depending on the month of pregnancy some meat soup but no meat. In the contemporary urban milieu this amounted to rice, wheat, broken wheat (preferably rice and parboiled rice, especially in the context of South India where it is the staple), milk, ghee, or clarified butter, some vegetables, only one of the common lentils (*mūng,* as it is easily digestible), a few select spices sparingly used, no tea, coffee, and nothing pungent; and for meat eaters, meat soup rather than flesh. Apart from the diet and drugs appropriate to each month, in the ninth month Teresa administered an unctuous enema made of oil and drugs with a "sweet taste" (*madhura rasa*), and tampons soaked in the same oil for oleation (*snehana*) of the uterus and the genital tract.

A regimen like this was premised on the fact that the predominant taste throughout the pregnancy ought to be sweet (*madhura rasa*).[38] The food ought to be palatable, easily digestible, and nourishing. Milk is nourishing, wholesome, and sweet, and to it are added drugs also of a sweet taste. *Madhura rasa* keeps *vāta* in check (for example cold food increases *vāta* as their properties are analogous); so do the ghee and the unctuous enema and oleation, as they have the properties of *snigdha* (unctousness) as opposed to *rūkṣa* (roughness), and of *uṣṇa* (hot, which of course depends on the oil and its mode of processing), as opposed to *śītala* (cool).

While all the three *doṣas* (roughly translated as humors, though this is contentious) are important, it is evident from the above that *vāta* is central. *Vāta* is responsible for all movement in the body (and pain). It is the only *doṣa* that moves, and hence among other things, is mobile, subtle, cold, dry, and rough: the entire diet and regimen are marshaled to counter these properties. There are five kinds of *vāta,* with one of them, the *Apāna-vāta,* being situated below the navel. *Apāna-vāta* is responsible for all movement in that region and its "natural" movement is downward. Its vitiation may lead to its obstruction or inversion (the *Apāna-vāta* begins to move in the wrong, upward direction) resulting in the impairment of all that normally moves downward in the area of the genitourinary tract, including the fetus.

Teresa and Urvashi (her associate and yoga teacher) also suggested an "exercise regimen" in the form of yoga. It was conceived by the trimester rather than by the month and began with a very mild set of exercises in the first trimester, as the fetus was not yet formed and was therefore prone to miscarriages. It was followed by a fuller course in the second trimester, which tapered off as the women reached full term. Since the yoga was taught as an adjunct to Ayurveda, Teresa's associate was acutely aware of *vāta-anulomana*: to keep the *vāta*, here the *Apāna-vāta*, moving in the right/downward direction so that the birth was easy and without any obstruction. The *āsana*s (postures) organized in a "parabolic" series first warmed up the body and allowed it to reach a peak—with the central set of exercises designed to ensure pelvic flexibility and ease of delivery. It ended with a set of sit-down breathing exercises (*prāṇāyāma*) that cooled the body, calmed the mind, and attempted to create a sense of equipoise. One of these exercises included meditating upon a visual image of the women's choice: one that filled them with peace and happiness and something whose attributes they thought the child should posses. The exercise was to first apprehend the object with eyes open and then to re-create and remember it with eyes shut. Vidya, who had used it rather effectively to control her blood pressure, told me that it was easier said than done, as it had required quite a bit of time and effort before she could master it.

The diet, drugs, and yoga were accompanied by a regimen that involved anointing the region from the waist to the knee with a generous amount of warm medicated oil half an hour before bathing, inviting the women to be calm and happy (worry and fear increases *vāta*), not to sleep during the day but to be reasonably active (excess activity vitiates *vāta*), and especially not to sleep after the midday meal, which is quite common in large parts of South Asia and especially in the warmer regions of southern India.[39]

Afternoon Sleep, Gestational Diabetes, and Morning Tea

Sangita also visited her gynecologist every month for her routine blood test, the occasional ultrasound scan, and for advice on her diet. In the seventh month she was diagnosed with gestational diabetes and sent off to a diabetologist. He decided that she didn't need any medication and passed her on to his dietician. The dietician drew up a chart during the course of which Sangita confessed to her that she was seeing an Ayurvedic doctor who, she said, had put her on a regimen and as part of it got her to start her mornings with *Jīraka-kaṣāyam* (an infusion of cumin, or "cumin tea").[40]

Sangita said, "the dietician, when she heard this, was cross and told me to stop all that nonsense and asked me to start my mornings with a cup of light black tea. I just switched off, and told myself that this is where I get off. I marched off the next morning to Teresa."

In a familiar scenario of disregarding the gynecologist's advice on just about everything, she appeared with the diet chart. According to Sangita, Teresa examined it and began to laugh, saying, "I'm sure you'll turn diabetic if you follow this." After a careful interrogation of her diet and eating habits, Teresa discovered that Sangita ate (or snacked) about six times a day and slept as if there was no tomorrow. She was annoyed, and said, "I thought I told you that you can't sleep during the day and especially not in the afternoon." Sangita denied this, to which Teresa replied, "well, I'm telling you now, if you sleep your baby will be a sleepyhead, and that's why you have put on so much weight and turned diabetic." She was then given some medicine for two weeks, at the end of which her sugar came down.

For Sangita's gynecologist (Madhu), sleep and weight were not a problem. Madhu had told her to get all the sleep she could, as she was unlikely to get much of it after the child was born; and as for weight, Madhu herself had put on twenty-four kilos, and now, said Sangita,

> There she was, slim and pretty! Madhu also told me to consume a lot of yoghurt and fruit, which, as you know, Teresa is dead set against. The only occasion where they both agreed was when it came to milk, and while for Teresa it was two glasses a day it was four for Madhu! I stuck to two. And probably the only time I did what Madhu asked of me was to have tetanus shots. It was to prevent infection during birth; and it made sense to me. But otherwise I followed Teresa's advice. But I wish Teresa were more communicative. She just presumes you know a lot of things, but you don't.

This reminded me of another of Teresa's patients, who had told me, "She'll say, 'Have some meat soup!' presuming I know how to make it." In opposition to this was Madhu the gynecologist who, said Sangita,

... was wonderful! Lovely manners, warm, and made you feel great. But you know they have no clue about diet and although I liked her, I didn't follow any of her advice. No folic acid after that initial panic, no vitamins or iron tablets or anything of that kind, and certainly no tea in the morning or large helpings of fruit and curd. But in all honesty I couldn't wholly follow Teresa either. She makes you go around in a tight little circle with rice, wheat, milk, ghee and some vegetable and a bit of spice, and that pomegranate. And she is aghast when we complain, and I'm sure all her patients complain bitterly. And her usual retort when we do complain is: isn't that enough, you could make a lot of things out of rice, wheat, milk, ghee, some vegetable and some spice!

This, I knew, was a widely shared sentiment: not just among women who had gone through their pregnancy with Teresa but all her patients, most of whom complained and pleaded with her to relax her dietary "restrictions," only to be sternly lectured by Teresa. But, as we saw, and as Teresa patiently pointed out to some of her patients, there is practically no distinction between food and medicine: food was often the cause of disease and hence it had to be "re-worked" if the disease was to be turned around, and carefully attended to if it was to be prevented. But surprisingly enough, many patients did not quite see it that way.[41]

Amniotic Fluid, Full Term, and the Caesarean

In her ninth month (on the fourth of October), Sangita went for a scan, precipitating a crisis. Madhu's mother-in-law, the matriarch and senior gynecologist, was there. The scan showed that her amniotic fluid count was a 9.5. "Under nine was a problem, and mine was a borderline case. The old fogey said she had to do a caesarean and fixed a tentative date for the seventh of October. I panicked. I called Teresa and she asked me not to panic and to hold on."

Unable to wait, her mind racing, she called Madhu and persuaded her to let her have a second opinion. She then went to the premier five-star hospital in Madras and, to her utter joy, came back with a reading of 11.5. The pathologist there told her not to panic and said that she could easily go through her full term and wait until the twenty-ninth of the month, which was her "due date." When she showed this rather triumphantly to the senior doctor, "the old fogey was furious," summoned Madhu (her daughter-in-law and junior gynecologist) and said that she would never have allowed the second opinion. She then told Sangita, "I'll wait at the latest till the eighteenth and if you don't go into labor by then, we'll admit you."

"On the seventeenth I went for my usual morning walk. I usually walk 2.5 km every morning. Sometime into my walk I started to panic. I was told to watch out for movement. But I couldn't detect any. I thought of Teresa and what she had repeatedly told me about how I shouldn't worry about term time and it could be well above nine months; and her saying, 'You wouldn't pluck a fruit before it is ripe.' But there was no movement; and there was a strange stillness in my belly. I had never quite felt like that."

Sangita then abandoned her walk and she and her husband rushed to the maternity clinic. She was examined, reassured of fetal movement, and told that there was a clear, discernible heartbeat coming from the womb. This was at seven in the morning. Only Madhu, the daughter-in-law and junior gynecologist, was there. The senior doctor on arrival immediately did another scan and found that Sangita's amniotic fluid reading had dropped to 3.5.

"She lost it. She immediately packed me off to another lab for a Doppler test to see if there was blood flow between mother and child. Oh, that was a horror! Had to wait for three hours, long queue, there were fifty people. It was like a factory—I don't want to go through it again! But the test showed there was flow, and also showed the baby had his cord around his neck."

When Sangita got back, she realized that they had decided to admit her and she was told in no uncertain terms that they were going to perform a caesarean on her the next morning.

Recounting this, she said, "I felt I was in prison; I always wanted Joy (her husband) by my side. They put me in a room, gave me lunch. Put me in a gown. Mom stayed the night. Before that I had worked on a film on hanging; about a revolutionary in prison. The hospital, the bath, the new clothes, it all felt the same. I consoled myself with the thought that in a while I would see the smiling face of my baby. They walk you into an operating room. Give you an injection like a lethal injection. Then they strap you. Strap your legs up. Talking to me . . . distracting me. A huge light when you look up. IV in bottles hung up. Then they come and I hear someone say spinal anesthesia.

137

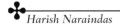

I had read somewhere that it is not good, so I tell them no spinal anesthesia but general anesthesia . . ."

Agency, Authority, and the Vade Mecum

Riessman (1993) has observed that individuals narrate particular experiences where there has been a breach between the ideal and the real and faced with the biographic disruption of chronic illness, reconstruct a coherent self in narratives. In Sangita's case the disruption between the ideal and the real was certainly not caused by a chronic illness but by amniotic fluid, medical technology, and the authority of the senior gynecologist, who decided that Sangita might not be able to carry her baby to full term and set a revised date, a date that hung over her head like the sword of Damocles. In Sangita's narrative, the ideal of a birth with Teresa, or at least of a normal birth with her gynecologist, had to be reconciled with the reality of a caesarean by the gynecologist. When she narrated her story to me, Sangita explicitly compared her plight to that of a revolutionary about to be executed for a crime, which shows just how strongly she felt that she had been deprived of meaningful agency, of control over her own body. Her last plea for general anesthesia, which may read as a last attempt to exercise her agency, is particularly ironic as general anesthesia is now passé and administered only in the case of an "emergency."[42]

All the women who, like Sangita, had been through the dual course between Teresa and their respective gynecologists were thus forced to negotiate between competing forms of "authoritative knowledge." Nearly all of them, and many of their husbands, agreed that this was their own predicament with their parents wary of the experiment and actually relieved that the birth was going to be in a hospital under *expert* supervision. One of them, Aditi, quite categorically told me, "My mother was happy that I had an episiotomy.[43] She had me at home and had a nightmare: her vagina had torn in the effort." Aditi, apart from the episiotomy, had a "normal delivery" and continues like Sangita to now negotiate between the gynecologist and Teresa for postpartum breast feeding and the pediatrician and Teresa for child care. Sangita, when she had a case of severe breast engorgement soon after her birth, first went to Madhu, who put her on drugs to reduce what she thought was excessive lactation, then went to Teresa who "steamed" her breast and gave her something to *regulate* her lactation. In a case of reverse "lying" to her "physician of choice," Sangita did not tell Teresa about her visit to the gynecologist. When I recounted this episode to Teresa, she said, "I now know why her milk supply came down drastically. She didn't tell me that she was on allopathic drugs and I thought that it was probably due to the drugs I had given her."

In all these narratives, what strikes one is the kind of choices that "lay" people are called upon to make and the kind of agency they are called upon to exercise in the face of expertise. While it is abundantly clear that agency is strongly exercised, the question is: what constrains it, or, what enables them to make the choices they make; and how, when, and why do they make them? One way in which the question of choice, agency, and expert authority has been addressed in the literature is by looking at doctor–patient interactions (hereafter DPI). Roughly four DPI models have been proposed: the paternalistic model where the doctor makes all the decisions; the interpretative model where the doctor elicits the values and needs of the patient and then makes the decision on his or her behalf; the shared decision-making model where, through dialogue and deliberation, doctor and patient arrive at a kind of consensus on the treatment and course of action; and finally the so-called informed decision making model, where the patient is presented with all the information and a set of choices on the basis of which *he or she* decides what to do.[44]   While the literature is clear that in any given case all four forms may coexist and slide into each other, and although we can quite easily see that all the four models are indeed at play in our narrative, the question of what cognitive, affective, economic, and social premises shape the decisions of patients, in situations where they are indeed able to exercise choice, is something that needs to be squarely addressed, theorized, and ethnographically worked out. Moreover, these lovely models simply fall apart in situations like this where all visits to the gynecologist are based on lies and, as it transpires, some visits to the Ayurvedic doctor, who is here the "primary physician," are also based on lies. And the primary physician, who is the main confidante of the patient, is unable to deliver the child, but nevertheless contests all that the gynecologist has to offer!

It is quite clear from our narrative that choice is most clearly exercised. While it is true that this "lay" choice is determined by social class, and even truer that the very desire to exercise choice is itself a class privilege (Lazarus 1994), we are left with the task of determining the mode and especially the content of this choice. Sangita's predicament is a variation of a trajectory that Lazarus describes for educated women in the United States who, even more than Sangita, often have a clear script for a "natural" childbirth experience in a hospital. But, as Lazarus shows, neither they, nor those in the health professions, including gynecologists, are always able to put this script into practice, not even in their own institutions. So-called contingencies, particularly as interpreted by an institutional and professional mandate, supervene. One gynecologist (and expectant mother) I interviewed in the United States had gone to great lengths to ensure that her script went according to plan. She had signed a written contract with a *doula* whose main job, apart from feet pressing and hand holding, was to constantly remind the birthing mother, in case she went into prolonged labor, not to succumb to an epidural if and when the certified nurse-midwife offered it to her. Her job was to remind the birthing woman, in her moment of agony and pain, and when her resolve was about to break, to "hang in there." It is eminently possible that her script, irrespective of her partner at her head and her *doula* at her feet, was ambushed. And knowing full well that it *may* be ambushed leads other women to plan and stage their deliveries entirely outside the portals of a hospital, and sometimes with dolphins in the high sea or in shark-infested lagoons, leading to a spectrum of possibilities (with their own waylaying, no doubt), whose epistemic and political premises form the backdrop to ontological enactments that one may not be able to capture through a disease/illness dichotomy a la Mol (2002).

While poor women, or rural women, may have a culture and worldview distinctly different from that of the gynecologist, in India the middle-class patient and doctor have often been to the same educational institutions and are literally "schooled" by social class into the same universe. In most instances, such patients and doctors share the same universe of meaning, and hence do not question the caesarean as medically dubious or unnecessary. In fact, for many well-to-do women, the caesarean, as I pointed out earlier, may well be a way of exercising choice against the ignominy of a vaginal birth and its associated "ritual pollution"; equally it may be a sign of social status, allowing these women and their in-laws to talk about the surgery, since vaginal birth cannot be so easily discussed, and/ or by believing that the caesarean is either painless (a widely held belief), or by consciously willing to exchange the aftermath of the pain of surgery for the pain of labor.[45] Hence, if the hospital birth, the C-section, and the episiotomy are treated as normative for middle-class women in India, the trajectories of women like Sangita are fraught. For her, unlike most of her peers, Dr. Spock's baby books (2004), which ostensibly functioned as an authoritative guide for a whole generation worldwide, are no longer quite the vade mecum;[46] and hospital birthing no longer has a taken-for-granted quality. What we witness instead is the shaping of her agency, or what Pickering (2008) would call a "dance of agency,"[47] between competing but *asymmetrical* forms of embodied authority made up of humans and nonhumans; ideas in the form of fragments of information through books, print and people; and, in "modern times," the next best or worst thing to the vade mecum: Google.com!

In some instances none of these "authoritative forms of knowledge" or fragments settle the matter. For Sangita, neither her gynecologist, nor Teresa, nor her family and friends could help with the next problem that arose. Having delivered her baby successfully, Sangita was unable to feed it.[48] The gynecologist offered her extremely uncomfortable "breast shields," about which Sangita said, "bloody hell, she didn't have a clue about breast shields. She got me to wear one of these, which is like the nipple of a feeding bottle . . . It was a nightmare. I went around with them for two weeks till someone got me some soft, foreign ones." Ultimately she was rescued by her maid, a mother of three young children, who showed her how to handle her breast so that she could feed her child.

Part of the negotiation that we witness here no doubt comes from a kind of agon: a contest between two "systems," with one of them, modern Ayurveda, a kind of a mongrel determined by at least a hundred years of shifting curricular history shaped by nationalist politics, colonialism, industrial pharmaceuticals, and global science. While it is true that all births in some senses may be problematic, arising from internal dissensions or points of view within a cosmogony or a milieu, here the form and nature of the action and choice by the expectant mother is conditioned by competing modes of *authority* and *expertise*. It is not merely, as Mol would have us believe, between the clinical and the pathological, between the point of view of disease and the point of view of illness or the point of view of the doctor and the point of view of the patient; or in another body of literature between the lifeworld of the doctor as opposed to the lifeworld of the patient and the dominance of the one over the other (Hak 2004; Mishler 2005), unless we "reduce" one of these modes of expert authority (Ayurveda) to culture and thus the life world of the patient, and elevate the other (obstetrics and gynecology) to science or nature, which is indeed the tacit frame of reference for much of medical anthropology, especially in the Third World. For many middle-class urban women nothing could be further from the truth, as they increasingly have no idea of the premises of Ayurveda through a form of ready and tacit socialization, which could then be seen as constituting their "culture." This is often compounded by the fact that their parents are often dead set against their purported choice—as we saw in the case of Sangita's father who, while he himself appeared to be seeing a "quack," accused the daughter of putting herself in the hands of a quack, who was a fully qualified physician and legally allowed to practice her science or craft, unlike *his* renegade physician turned *siddha vaidya,* who lived on coconut water and a lump of clay once a day. And despite *his* "quack" having *cured* him of his diabetes, he did not want his daughter to go anywhere near an Ayurvedic physician, for something as *grave* as childbirth.

Hence, what we have here are (at least) two competing approaches to pregnancy, based on competing nosologies and ontologies, asymmetrically related to each other at this particular historical juncture, inviting either approbation or guilt for those exercising a choice. The exercising of this choice is not the end but the beginning of a minefield that the patient is now called upon to traverse and negotiate, with no vade mecum at hand. And vade mecums are cardinal as they offer a script, but any breach of this script entails the risk of it going hopelessly wrong as it could have for Sangita.[49]

Nosopolitics: Proliferating Epistemologies

It is evident that this chapter is not only about exercising choice but also about what happens *after* one has exercised it. In other words it is not about claims to an "easy" pluralism, where patients readily and seamlessly choose "all therapies at once," are able to shuttle between seemingly different *nosologies* with their attendant epistemologies and ontologies, and readily translate between them, or hold together things that may be contradictory (even though all of these things may sometimes happen). What we witness here is the *experiential consequence* of this shuttling, which may have enormous consequences for the protagonists. Rejecting folic acid, with spina bifida as a possible consequence, foregoing the dietician's advice with the prospect of the diabetes getting worse, having a "tetanus shot" as "it makes sense" and prevents the prospect of tetanus, "succumbing" to a Doppler test and "agreeing" to a caesarean so as to give birth "safely"—all these are the consequences that follow (or do not follow) the making of particular choices.

In this instance, it is clear that such *choosing* may not be easily captured by the distinction between the disease of the doctor and the illness of the patient and its several homologues, which may be understood by the rather apt phrase coined by Mol, that we are confronted by "more than one but less than many" (Mol 2002). While Mol rightly and courageously breaches the presupposition of a single disease entity by showing that the disease of the clinician and the disease of the pathologist are not the same (and if we add the illness—nay disease—of the patient, we get an even more complex picture), it still presupposes a fragmented but single (?) episteme, whose ontological enactments, depending on the site and the situation, produce more than one therapeutic format, which too may have, and in fact does have, consequences. If we extend this to our current case, we can argue that there is, for example, a division among pediatricians, geriatricians, and general physicians on the question of folic acid. The pediatricians cannot have enough of it and are unhappy with the amount of folic acid in fortified bread as laid down by the FDA. While they want more, the geriatricians want none of it, as it is bad news for the geriatric population and osteoporosis. The general physicians are of the opinion that one can get enough folic acid from eating the right type of food and fortifying bread is unnecessary.[50] Each of these is different from saying that one does not need folic acid at all; or that spina bifida, or tetanus, as nosological categories do not exist, as they may not in Ayurvedic nosology. In this instance we may have to entertain the possibility that there are "more than one" and this more than one are *many* rather than "less than many that hang together"; in other words, we do have more than one disease, or more than one patient, or more

143

than one prospective mother, all of whom do *not* "hang together."
Or we may have to say that there is one person(?) with several kinds
of pregnancies, or several kinds of invaginations, that is, if it were
possible to use the word invagination merely descriptively. Hence,
it may better to say with several ways of construing the *difficulty*
with postpartum breast feeding:[51] one Ayurvedic, one gynecolog-
ical, and a third that we have glossed by reducing it to the "experiential practice" of the maid who resolves the problem, thereby
doing injustice to what may well stem from another epistemology
that has no ready codex, or one that we—and who is that we?—are
not aware of and hence suffers the fate of an *ontological enactment*
sans a codex.[52]

It is imperative, given the above elucidation, that we move on to
consider the possibility of several and at times competing nosologies, based on competing epistemologies, in whose shadow agency is
exercised and ontological enactments occur, leading to a blurring if
not a mangling of therapies by patients, whose *consequences* may not
be pretty if they result in deformed bodies or babies. These prolif-
erations of bodies and bodies of knowledge seem particularly acute
currently as "alternative" epistemologies, which are themselves part
symptom of internal dissensions in allopathy, as they, especially in
the case of pregnancy, have partly engendered these debates and
dissensions.[53] Having engendered them, they step into these ongoing dialogues and transform them and are in turn transformed by
them for they too are fractured, and have been fractured and recast
by allopathy and a materialist metaphysics. This is evident from the
narrative recounted here as the patient/person/prospective mother is
caught in this maelstrom, and her very desire to exercise choice may
be read as the symptom of a maelstrom on the question of pregnancy
and childbirth.[54]

But such a maelstrom should not blind us to the analytical distinction between competing ways of construing the world based on
different metaphysical premises, which in turn lead to competing
ways of construing diseases, competing theories of nutrition, and
competing pharmacopeias, where therapeutic substances in one are
banned substances in another, some of which are regularly administered by Teresa to her patients, causing much consternation and
debate within her own fraternity of physicians for whom the biomedical pharmacopeia is often the norm. To not acknowledge this

nosopolitics is to annul the possibility of other kinds of Beings, and of other ways of being in the world.

Acknowledgments

This chapter owes its existence to the two principal dramatis personae in this article: Teresa and Sangita (pseudonyms, as are all the other names in the article). I would like to thank them for their warmth, generosity, time, and unstinted support; and the wonderful support and generosity of Teresa's family and her colleagues, especially Urvashi the cofounder and principal yoga teacher/therapist at the clinic; Teresa's husband who forever kept us in good humor; and Teresa's therapists, interns, support staff, and patients, who appear here through pseudonyms. The chapter equally owes thanks to all the persons and institutions in the United States, especially Paul and Adrian (and some in Germany and the U.K., including Deepa and Krishna Kumar) who were kind enough to entertain and enable my research, and who shared so much of themselves with me. This was especially the case with the lay midwives in the United States, who slowly, and initially reluctantly, came out of the woodwork to talk to me, as lay midwifery was illegal in this state. It is evident, given the amount of time this has taken to see the light of day, that I have accumulated more debts then I can possibly recall, including successive classes of students in three universities where I have tried these ideas out, some of whom went out of their way and played an enabling role, including introducing me to midwives. Several people (apart from Teresa and her husband who have kindly read several drafts) have been kind enough to read earlier drafts of this chapter (Polit, Chakravarthy, Mukherjee, Yadav, Ahlin, and Gopalan), including the three anonymous referees to this volume, whose diligent and thought-provoking comments have been helpful in revising it, as have the comments and scrupulous reading by my co-editors, especially Bo Sax for his selfless and repeated reading of the chapter. It has also benefited from the readings of Ananda Samir Chopra, fellow traveler and collaborator at the Karl Jaspers Centre of the University of Heidelberg, which through its Cluster of Excellence awarded me a Joint-Appointment Professorship (2008–2012), thus enabling subsequent research and writing of this piece. It has been a pleasure to work with Johannes and Bo on this volume and this chapter owes a lot to their presence, as it does to the constant presence of Nupur Barua, who has been instrumental in seeing it through.

Notes

1. For instance, according to the German *Statistisches Bundesamt* (National Census Bureau), there were 667,464 children born (registered) in Germany in 2009, of which 656,265 births or 98.32 percent were born in hospitals. The other 11,199 children were born in out-of-hospital facilities (home, birthing center or *Geburtshaus*, and doctor's practice). The majority

of out-of-hospital births took place in *Geburtshäusern*, which was closely followed by home births. Only a fraction took place in doctors' practices (QUAG 2012).

2. These are the official statistics, which may well be belied by empirical research.

3. MacKinnon and McIntyre's paper (2006), which is on the recent "constitution of preterm labor risk in pregnancy," alludes to risk in pregnancy in general and sees preterm labor risk as a continuation of this trend. For another interesting piece on the general history of risk in medicine, see the recent article by Timmermann (2011), which recounts the adoption into both East and West Germany of the postwar construction of risk in American medicine, built primarily around diet and cardiovascular diseases. One of the critiques of risk that came up in the 1970s in West Germany was the argument that the notion of risk leads to the collapsing of prevention and treatment, where risk begins to be seen as a "cause" of disease and hence may be prevented by treating it. In other words, risk is another instance, if not a fundamental instance, of medicalization, "as the risk factor concept appeared to medicalize people who did not necessarily feel sick when physiological parameters such as blood pressure or blood cholesterol went above a more or less arbitrary threshold" (Timmermann 2011: 170). While pregnancy may be a prime case in point, "risk" may have a much longer genealogy than postwar American medicine, as is presumably the case with breast cancer (Jasen 2002). We must be wary of positing that other historical periods and cultures did not see pregnancy as being "risky." But we must be equally careful not to read the past and the Other from the standpoint of the present and the West; as what risk means, and how it is embedded in a sociotechnical fabric, is something that needs careful investigation. Hence, presumably among the Kalahari, a woman was encouraged to undertake the "risky" venture of giving birth on her own in the bush, without anyone attending on her (Biesele 1997). Such an "unassisted birth" was especially "encouraged" after the first pregnancy. The Ju/'hoansi of the Kalahari clearly saw pregnancy as not only "risky" but as a wager against death, quite like hunting or going into a shamanistic trance. Like both these male activities, the "solo" pregnancy was seen as being spiritually transformative and conferred a superior status on the successful mother (Biesele 1997). While this may well be true, and offers a different perception of the risk associated with pregnancy, one is struck by the fact that this article, with the rather apt title of "an ideal of unassisted birth," was placed by the editors (Davis-Floyd and Sargent 1997) at the end of their collection. It thus appears as the apotheosis of a counternarrative to the medicalization of pregnancy, namely the "rugged individualism" of the Kalahari woman, which in turn finds resonance today in seeing the "natural/home birth" as both an aesthetic and moral adventure (see note 7 below for a current resonance and note 53 for a counter to this "counternarrative") of the contemporary (Western?) woman and her "rugged individualism," along with the "spiritually transformative potential" of pregnancy. Hence, it is none too

surprising that what are called complementary and alternative medicine in general, of which home/natural births may be seen a subspecies, have a strong aesthetic, moral, and spiritual strand (cf. Kirmayer, this volume and Warrier, this volume).

4. For an early critique of this term, see Hardin (1968). This is a central phrase in the current American "pro-life" (Hardin in 1968 calls them the "prohibitionists") discourse, where the "unborn child" is constructed as the doctor's "second patient," leading to the reframing of the contemporary debate in terms of a "maternal–fetal conflict." For a good example of a "prohibitionist/pro-life" documentary film that plays this up, see *The Silent Scream.*

5. See note 37 for an elaboration and for how technology may, in the same breath, both mitigate and exacerbate risk.

6. One tends to agree with Davis-Floyd insofar as she turns the tables by calling "obstetric procedures" rituals. What this does, however, is to (a) retain the dichotomy between ritual and nonritual and, more importantly, (b) possibly prevent us from seeing that what have hitherto been called rituals elsewhere may, in the context of "healing," be "medically" efficacious procedures. I use the word medically deliberately, as these rituals may ostensibly be in a religious setting, and the "nosology" in such a setting may, for example, be seen as a "demonology." Several of the chapters in this volume grapple precisely with this phenomenon, thus inviting us to rethink these boundaries. I have elsewhere shown (Naraindas 1998, 2003a) that there may exist a strict isomorphism between the protocols of "worship" and the protocols of "medicine." This was/is the case with the procedures adopted for "smallpox" in India, where what one "does" to the deity is isomorphic to what one does to the patient; and where the patient in fact is the deity as the smallpox deity is *in* the patient.

7. I have a long narrative of an Austrian doctor in Germany who gave birth in the Caribbean on a quasi-private island with a lagoon, after abandoning the possibility of a birth on a more remote one as it was shark infested. This one too ran the *risk* of sharks being attracted by the blood, but she took the plunge, as there was help at hand, including the possibility of summoning a helicopter to transport her to a hospital in the case of an emergency. The second birth was in a tub in her garden.

8. I was under the impression that the word *nosopolitics,* which in fact is the title of another article of mine (Naraindas 2014), was a neologism coined by me! It readily suggested itself to me as it is one of the central arguments here as it is in the other piece and arises from what I allude to here as multiple and competing nosologies and their *experiential consequences.* But it turns out that Foucault has used this term (presumably only in his 1980 article) in the context of the emergence of a medical market in the context of the politics of health in eighteenth-century Europe, where he says: "The sudden importance assumed by medicine in the eighteenth century originates at the point of intersection of a new 'analytical' economy of assistance with the emergence of a general 'police' of health. The new nosopolitics inscribes the specific question of the sickness of the poor with

the general problem of the health of populations and makes the shift from the narrow context of charitable aid to the more general form of a 'medical police' imposing its constraints and dispensing its services" (Foucault 1980: 171). While Foucault has been central to my work (Naraindas 1996) in the past and continues to be so, I believe my use of this neologism in the context of competing epistemic or *therapeutic* "systems," although it may have a family resemblance to Foucault's use, indexes, as is evident, something quite different. I use the word therapeutic as opposed to "medical" systems, as the site of curing (I again choose not to use word *healing* deliberately, although I have done so elsewhere in the article) may well be in what appears to be a "religious" context, as is the case with several of the chapters here.

9. Several of the chapters in this volume (Basu, Quack, Sax and Bhaskar) deal with these seemingly marginalized systems, practices, or facets, which have no state backing and are often under threat.

10. Many of the ethnographies in this volume testify to the existence of these other nosologies (even if the concept is seemingly absent in their writing and the authors do not directly address it) along with their attendant therapeutic strategies. This is particularly "vibrant" and relatively "unsullied" when it comes to "mental illness" (this may not be the native term), and often the "difficulty," or *saṅkaṭ* (to use one of several terms, depending on which part of South Asia one is in), experienced by the person may not be on the register of "illness," or illness alone, or, as is often the case in these chapters, they may lie on the register of "possession" and "exorcism," all rather problematic terms, which I will take up toward the end of the chapter. It is important to note from the studies assembled here that this is the case across religion, region, caste, and social class, and between "textual" and "oral" traditions.

11. Lay midwives in the United States are midwives who are not part of the formal hospital system. Their status varies depending on the regulations of the state where they are practicing. "As of July 1987, ten states have prohibitory laws, five states have grandmother clauses authorizing practicing midwives under repealed statutes, five states have enabling laws which are not used, and ten states explicitly permit lay midwives to practice. In the twenty-one remaining states, the legal status of midwives is unclear" (Butter and Kay 1988: 1161). In May 2008, a Pennsylvania court in Lancaster County (which has a significant Amish population) kept open this ambiguity by saying that a lay midwife who helped in delivery was not practicing medicine. It transpires that "lay midwives attended almost fifty percent of the 3,481 out-of-hospital births in the state in 2004" (Medical News Today, Nursing/Midwifery News, 2008).

12. All these terms—midwife, *dai* (usually translated as midwife), and TBAs—are problematic to say the least. For a review of this literature and the politics of these terms see Pigg (1997) and Naraindas (2009).

13. Despite the promotion of this *solution,* according to the National Family and Health Statistics (NFHS) of the government of India for 1992–1993,

the rate of infant mortality both at home and in an institutional setting was exactly the same for rural India at 48.4 deaths per thousand; for urban India it was marked by a small difference—34.1 deaths per thousand at home as against 31.3 in public health facilities (Haq 2008: 27).

14. In the United States it was 19.8 percent in 2000 (Selvaraj et al. 2007: 11). It is evident that what is true of India may well be true of the Third World as a study of all vaginal deliveries performed in 1997 and 1998 at the University of Benin Teaching Hospital, Benin City, Nigeria, found that episiotomy rates were 46.6 percent among all deliveries, and in the case of first pregnancies they were as high as 87.4 percent (Otoide et al. 2000). As far as Europe is concerned the episiotomy rates in 2004 were: Germany: 30.8 percent, Denmark: 9.7 percent, Netherlands: 24.3 percent, U.K. England: 16.4 percent, U.K. Wales: 14.2 percent, U.K. Scotland: 21.1 percent Available at http://www.europeristat.com/bm.doc/european-perinatal-health-report.pdf. Accessed 28 December 2011.

15. But Pamela Stone (2009) quotes much larger figures for the United States, and also offers an interesting historical reading of the caesarean. In Germany every third birth (or 31.3 percent of births) in 2009 was a caesarean birth. In Denmark it could be as low as 10 percent, and in the U.K. it could be about 24 percent.

16. For a case of the promotion of hospital births in the making and raising of a new worker and new citizen in communist China of the 1950s, see Goldstein (1998), and for a case of "annulling" child spacing and the promotion of bottle feeding in a bid to make the Congolese have more babies so as to breed captive labor in a mining town under a colonial regime in the Belgian Congo, see Hunt (1988). It appears that science and medicine often transcend political differences, leading, in some fundamental ways, to the near universal marking and making of modern subjects through particular biopolitical practices: a perfect index of the shaping of both a cognitive and bodily disposition, or a "habitus," that fashions a brave new world for its subjects from the age of five if not three. Such "public health goods" are so universal, so successful and hence so sacrosanct, that the WHO and UNICEF are periodically able to broker cease-fire vaccination campaigns between warring factions like the Sri Lankan state and the Liberation Tigers of Tamil Elam (LTTE), where child soldiers are vaccinated for polio during a two-day cease-fire, only to be immediately redeployed in the war. The global eradication of polio (as is the case with the global eradication of many other things, including, in the context of this chapter, the eradication of home births in the third world currently promoted by the same UNICEF) is so paramount that it is able to repeatedly punctuate civil wars worldwide to vaccinate unvaccinated children, even if they may be killed the next day! The message seems to be that such "public health goods" are good enough even to trump war, even if momentarily. For a reading, however, of what these campaigns may mean for global public health institutions in terms of their institutional mandates, how they are economically crucial for disease surveillance organizations of First World countries like

the United States and how the overwhelming financial burden is borne by Third World states, with the Third World thus offering the First World a financial gift *in perpetuity*, see Naraindas (2003b, 2007).

17. These rituals, or sacraments, are quite cardinal and are among the central reasons for a home birth among the poor (Haq 2008; Naraindas 2009). Other equally important reasons stem from the fact that the poor are treated badly in public health institutions and are ready sites for family planning programs where, among other things, contraceptives are inserted or administered without their consent (Van Hollen 2003), and, as it transpires, not necessarily any safer.

18. For a good account of this interplay between current commodity consumption and a status economy in the context of childbirth, see Van Hollen (2003), especially her chapter on the pregnancy "rituals" of *cimantam* in Tamil Nadu, which shows that the interplay increasingly cuts across social classes. Equally interesting is the chapter on invoking *vali* (pain, suffering) by poor women and semirural women, where "*vali*/pain" during childbirth has a very different valence (ironically transformed by Pitocin) than it purportedly does (by implication) for middle-class women. Finally, a sustained reading of her work, on what *vali*/pain comes to mean to her *during* fieldwork, and *after* the loss of her own child, which she addresses in the appendix, makes for fascinating reading, leading to a kind of "before and after engagement with pain" that resonates with the politics of childbirth in note 53.

19. The current "secular" variant of this "auspicious time" was the desire of middle-class women (reported in several Indian English-language newspapers) to give birth (and thus have a "unique" birth date) on 12 December 2012 (or 12.12.12), while elsewhere others (especially evangelical groups in the United States) geared up (with bow and arrow) for the apocalypse (also reported, with pictures, in the same newspapers)!

20. For a classic satire of "disease snobbery," see the essay "Selected Snobberies" by Aldous Huxley (1966).

21. As Bhasin et al. (2007) say, "Caesarean section is a lucrative surgical procedure and therefore commercial interest may well have been the motive force behind the exceptionally high rate and many of these procedures may not have been to the benefit to the mother or fetus." But despite the critique, nothing by way of an alternative (to a hospitalized delivery) is remotely suggested by the authors.

22. It is instructive that despite very "widespread talk" among prospective mothers in Germany about going to a birthing center (*Geburtshaus*), most do not. Anthropologist colleagues at Heidelberg were surprised to learn that 98 percent of births in Germany were in a hospital. Most had presumed it would be far less. Perhaps it is only women of a certain social class or educational level in Germany who actively consider alternative birthing institutions (but usually do not utilize them).

23. Women seeing the nurse-midwife often downloaded a "twenty-point natural birth" checklist from the internet and took it with them for their first

consultation. See, for example, Angela England's (2007) blog on the internet for a set of "twenty" questions that one may ask an obstetrician about pregnancy and childbirth.

24. "In response to a push for more 'natural' birth events, many hospitals now offer more modern options for low-risk births, often known as family-centered care. These may include private rooms with baths (birthing suites) where women can labor, deliver, and recover in one place without having to be moved" (http://kidshealth.org/parent/system/doctor/birth_centers_hospitals.html).

25. This would be a good example of what in current popular marketing parlance would be called a win-win situation: the woman, like before, is delivered *of* the child *by* the obstetrician (passive woman and delivering doctor) and, at the same time, now actively delivers the child (active woman and active doctor/midwife). This is evidently a response to the large body of literature that has shown how the lithotomic or supine position, by defying gravity, is a problematic position (Bhardwaj et al. 1995; Gupta and Nikoderm 2000; Odent 2001; DiFranco et al. 2007) and to the studies documenting the advantages that accrue from the "upright or squatting position" (Bhardwaj et al. 1995; Mathews et al. 2005).

26. *Doula* is the Greek word for a woman servant. Today it has come to mean a woman who specializes in helping a pregnant woman and her family through the childbearing year.

27. In Germany, 15.6 percent of the 10,669 out-of-hospital births in 2010 were transferred to a hospital, according to personal correspondence with Christine Loytved.

28. For these outcome statistics on out-of-hospital births for 2010 in Germany see Loytved (2012).

29. I visited two *Geburtshäuser* in Kassel (one in a spiritual commune that had four different birthing rooms, each named after a natural element), and interviewed midwives and mothers who had delivered there. In the U.K. I visited a hospital in Norwich, and conducted a long interview with the midwife who attended my niece during birth. My thanks to them, as well as to the *Geburtshaus,* the commune, and the midwives and the mothers in Kassel.

30. In the last few years, she has "graduated" to delivering children in her clinic thus largely obviating the kind of narrative that this chapter analyzes. I say "largely" as the particular kind of movement between her and a gynecologist, if at all, will need empirical investigation.

31. There are interesting parallels between her situation and that of the licensed midwives in the United States. Like licensed midwives in those American states where they are legal, the *vaidya,* too, is legally allowed to practice. But her contestation of the modern hospital is akin to those states in the United States where lay midwifery is illegal and where these midwives are not formally and legally wired to the hospital system.

32. In fact she is also constrained by her institutional training. "Modern doctors of traditional medicine" (an oxymoron) are taught a combination of

Ayurveda and biomedicine (allopathy as it is called in India) with a kind of amalgam where, among other things, surgical procedures are invariably through an internship in allopathic hospitals, including, and especially for, obstetrics and gynecology. This turns them into "second class citizens" during this internship, quite like their degree, which is a "second class degree" compared to the allopathic degree (Naraindas 2006). One symptom of this is indexed by the two renderings of the degree that is conferred on them, namely BAMS. This acronym is rendered as either a Bacherlor in Ayurveda, Medicine, and Surgery, or as a Bachelor in Ayurvedic Medicine and Surgery. But the syllabus, irrespective of these two renderings is an amalgam and, as I have called it elsewhere, a Creole (Naraindas 2014).

33. This is based on fieldwork done from 2001 to 2003. She subsequently began to deliver children (see note 30). But she has delivered only around ten children or so in the last six years, testimony to the fact that unlike the rest of her bustling practice, women opting to deliver with her are absurdly few, while the numbers of women who see her along with a gynecologist during their pregnancy is much greater.

34. This seems to be the case in the formal degree-granting institutions, which is why the BAMS graduates have to often intern in allopathic institutions, with obstetrics being a good case in point.

35. A woman who reincarnates, she claimed, an ancient figure—the *bogar*. The *bogar* is considered to be one of the eighteen *siddhars* (alchemists, mystics, healers) in the Tamil tradition, from whom the current *siddha* system of Tamil medicine is presumably derived (cf. White 1996, on Indian alchemy and the *siddha* tradition, and Weiss 2009 for the Tamil medical *siddha* tradition). This particular *bogar,* she said, had either physically traveled or had done astral travel to China and had learned medicine there.

36. I learned after talking to about 500 patients over three years that this kind of behavior is commonplace. Patients may offer themselves and not their children if they are skeptical; or if they are "converted" then, as neophytes, will *only* give Ayurvedic medicines to their children (especially infants), while subjecting themselves to "strong" and "dangerous" allopathic medicines. For these neophytes, at least their children should "return" and be resocialized into the old-new church. Others will parcel out different parts of their bodies, or different kinds of illnesses, to different kinds of therapies. We will see some of this in the narrative to follow.

37. It dawned on me that these attendant social technologies (for finding partners for example), seemingly available in a privileged lily-white university town, may be sadly lacking either in a black neighborhood hospital, or most certainly in India, thus leading to an enormous gulf between what a medical technology (usually more easily available) may accomplish and its resultant "failure" in the social world. This became doubly evident after the "working-class" prospective "spina bifida mother" left, as both the nurse and especially the pediatrician, were faintly disapproving of the young woman nursing the ambition of having a child she "could not possibly rear." This was followed by a moral commentary on the underclass and its

strange behavior (like rural farmers with poor social skills importing Russian mail-order brides), which brought much grief to its subjects, quite like the "spaced out" spina bifida mother (she turned burgers in a McDonald's, was all of twenty, and seemed to be in a daze and not quite there, which may have been because of the prognosis), who, without anyone quite stating it, was seen as being responsible for the spina bifida, and, to boot, had the audacity to entertain the possibility of having the child. I could well imagine what was in store for her and her possible child in this *privileged* little university town. But it is important to note that we *should not* therefore assume that a moral compunction to either abort or have a differently abled child, enabled by technology, is felt acutely only by the underclass (or imputed to them), because of a possible "lack of access to privileges." It is, I believe, felt by all women (which is why Sangita picked up her perfectly healthy child and began to examine its spine), and a refusal to address this (I attempt this elsewhere) black-boxes the technology and places it beyond moral scrutiny.

38. One of the six tastes (*rasas*), each of which either increases or decreases one or two of the three *doṣas*. The entire pharmacopeia and all foods are classified according to the six *rasas*, which have a mathematically worked out formal relationship to the six seasons, the three *doṣas*, the seven *dhātus* (body tissues), the five senses, the five elements, and so on. I am merely *indicating*, through the above, the logic of the regimen (cf. Zimmermann 1987 for a textual elucidation).

39. Food and sleep each on their own increase *kapha-doṣa*, and the two together are deadly as *kapha*, body weight and body fat are intimately tied to each other. Hence, no siesta (common in this part of the world) except a very short one in the height of summer (there are reasons for the choice of season) is recommended. The exceptions are infants, the very old, and the ill. The importance of this will brought home in the next episode of the narrative.

40. A *kaṣāyam* is a decoction (where the herb is cooked in water for a while, that is, the amount of water is reduced to either one-quarter or one-eighth), while an infusion (where the herb is not *cooked* in water) would be a *phāṇṭa* (when prepared with hot water) or *hima* (cold infusion). But in the clinical setting the word used was *kaṣāyam*, which is the generic term in the text for the above processes.

41. For an interesting commentary on the importance of food and health, see Alter's *The Wrestler's Body* (1992), where the wrestler is made to offer a commentary on the utterly fraught nature of food in India. Such a medico–moral commentary, however, is by no means limited to wrestlers. It is in fact ubiquitous for the urban generation over sixty years of age, and also for younger people in the countryside (although this can vary dramatically by class, caste, region, and education). But for the younger, urban generation fashioned by a modern and universal curriculum, food appears to be largely innocuous. Unless their dietician, fashion, or health magazine says so, anything may be eaten at anytime and anywhere, quite like the contemporary

153

*super*market where *all things are available in all seasons in all places.* The ideas of Teresa, for whom food was both "poison" and "medicine," would have warmed the hearts of a wrestling Guru. These competing theories of nutrition (biomedical doctors often call them nutrition as opposed to superstition, while anthropologists often say nutrition as opposed to cultural beliefs, which is far more insidious) are often dramatically played out in the hospital postpartum, with grandmothers, mothers, and mothers-in-law quarreling with the gynecologist on what the new mother could and could not be fed; the quarrel often starts with colostrums, seen to be rich in antibodies by doctors, but invariably (not always) seen as being utterly indigestible, and hence harmful, by the family.

42. See Anaesthesiology Info (2002).
43. Woolley (1995: 806), in a critical review of episiotomy says:
    NTX "the professional literature on the benefits and risks of episiotomy was last reviewed critically in 1983, encompassing material published through 1980. The purpose of this paper is to review the evidence accumulated since then. It is concluded that episiotomies prevent anterior perineal lacerations (which carry minimal morbidity), but fail to accomplish any of the other maternal or fetal benefits traditionally ascribed, including prevention of perineal damage and its sequel, prevention of pelvic floor relaxation and its sequel, and protection of the newborn from either intracranial hemorrhage or intra-partum asphyxia. In the process of affording this one small advantage, the incision substantially increases maternal blood loss, the average depth of posterior perineal injury, the risk of anal sphincter damage and its attendant long-term morbidity (at least for midline episiotomy), the risk of improper perineal wound healing, and the amount of pain in the first several postpartum days."
    (cf. Selvaraj et al. 2007; Naraindas 2008).
44. This, as Wirtz, Cribb, and Barber (2006: 118) point out, is different from the "legal" requirement of "informed consent," where the patient's consent is solicited for a course of action that has been decided upon by the doctor. This is not to say that it may not resemble the informed decision-making model in some or many instances. But as the authors quite rightly point out, it is important to make the distinction.
45. The worst but not at all unusual case seems to be a long and difficult labor with the help of epidural that "fails" (the cervix not dilating, the baby has its cord around its neck, it is a breech presentation, the labor is too long even with Pitocin, and so forth . . . I have heard each of these stories from women) resulting in a caesarean.
46. Like Gideon's Bible (the "original" vade mecum) in the top drawer of United States motels, put there to assuage the temptation and doubt of the traveling salesperson, or *The Anglo-Indian's Vademecum* (Hull and Mair 1878) born of white anxiety in the tropics (Naraindas 1996).
47. I am borrowing from Pickering (2008) what appears to be an apt phrase that seems appropriate for the context. Its use here may have more than a mere family resemblance to Pickering's use, insofar as the "dance" here,

as in the case with him, certainly involves the play between the human and the nonhuman in determining Sangita's trajectory, thought it is also a different kind of dance produced by competing forms of expertise, knowledge, authority, etc., within a larger canvas of historically contingent and construed "risk." Apart from that, while I am in general agreement about Pickering's motives and what he calls "ontology of becoming," as opposed to that familiar *dualism* that this volume too wrestles with, I am ambivalent about several other things he has to say.

48. It seemed like a mild case of "invagination" that one out of five women seem to suffer from. And there appears to be some debate on whether this is exacerbated if not "caused" by a C-section given the fact that women (also based on several women's personal testimony) are often unable to feed their babies immediately after a caesarean birth with any sense of comfort (they are, among other things, often unable to even turn on their sides to feed the newborn). This may be further compounded by the fact (though not in this case) that women at particular historical moments were discouraged from breast feeding and asked to bottle-feed the child (a practice that evidently reappears on the firmament under different guises, cf. the article by Hunt on the turn to bottle feeding in the Belgian Congo to induce child spacing in note 16 above), which in turn may have led to the worsening of the condition rather than resolving it, as postpartum breast feeding often resolves forms of invagination. In the same breath, a swing in the other direction of the *absolute* necessity to breast-feed the child may result in forms of panic, anxiety, guilt, and inadequacy!

49. The woman's magazine in particular, and Q & A's to doctors, psychiatrists, beauticians, dieticians, fashion designers, and fitness experts in newspapers and magazines, are just some of the burgeoning vade mecums at hand, which constantly tell people what to do, and when and how. In the Indian women's magazines, apart from "do's and don'ts" from the time you wake up to the time you go to bed, the vade mecum also offers tantalizing possibilities of breach, for example through richly elaborated narratives of adultery, only to make sure that they all end in tragedy. The message is that adultery does not pay. Imagine the lifelong *double* guilt if Sangita's *breach* of the received script (of "sleeping" with the *other* doctor/vaidya) had had gone wrong!

50. We can multiply this ad infinitum on how there can be four different ways of addressing a knee replacement by four different subspecialties in knee replacement surgery, or how interventional radiologists "see" adenomyosis differently from gynecologists and so on. Here Mol's work is cardinal as she shows how all these different "practices" produce different kind of bodies that are then articulated and speak, or made to speak, to each other. One could certainly, if one houses an Ayurvedic physician inside an allopathic hospital, perhaps then extend the analysis, by "reducing" Ayurveda to another "practice" (though this is moot). But that is evidently not the case here, especially given the contestation at work and the *experiential consequences* that follow. But we can also do the opposite and extrapolate from the ethnography *here* to interrogate whether different disciplinary

practices, even within a seemingly "single episteme" that constitutes an allopathic hospital of the kind that Mol describes, do indeed hang together. We can then go on to further ask whether some of the mortality and perhaps a substantial part of the morbidity, which is seen to result from iatrogenesis, is a consequence of things *not* "hanging together."

51. Quite like the difficulty, as I pointed out earlier, and to which I promised to return, with rendering the word *saṅkaṭ* (difficulty, problem) as one that is only on the register of illness; or the difficulties that one gets into by calling it possession (or any such term), all or some of which may already, given the history of these terms and they way they are embedded in both anthropological and medical literature, may prejudge the case, with the best example being the word possession that up to the Disease and Statistical Manual (DSM) IV, of the American Psychiatric Association (APA), is classified as a pathology. In other words, "my" *saṅkaṭ* in "your" register is possession and hence a pathology! This is notwithstanding the several distinctions that the DSM IV may make about different kinds of possession and how some, especially those in a "religious context," may be excluded from being pathologies (cf. Smith 2006)

52. See Kalpana Ram (2009) in the context of pregnancy, where she says that looking for a codex is an anthropological preoccupation, and how Leonnere Manderson, again in the context of pregnancy in Malaysia, is seen to construct a codex out of what are called "practices," which as Ram quite rightly points out follows different norms to be a repository in individuals and communities, and where apprenticeship is the usual pedagogic form. We can multiply this from the history of anthropology and talk about boat building, bridge building, etc., all of which are "practices" in several parts of the world before the anthropologist comes along and "builds" a codex; or as was presumably the case with church fathers in several parts of the world, a Latin codex either supplants (quite like the anthropological codex?), or is the only surviving testimony to the existence of native codices that went up in flames during an auto-da-fé. The best example of three codices (or three copies of a single codex), purportedly inspired by the Devil, that survived an auto-da-fé by the Friar Diego de Landa (1524–1579), are the Mayan ones at Dresden, Paris, and Madrid.

53. For an evenhanded review of these dissensions and the politics of childbirth, see the article by Beckett (2005). Beckett attempts to take on board current feminist critics of the so-called natural birth movement, whose presumed advocacy of the embracing of pain and prolonged labor has led some feminists to call them "birth junkies" (2005: 260) and has led "one feminist critic" to argue that "the 'natural' philosophy espoused in an alternative birth center is as tyrannical and prescriptive as the medical model, but pretends not to be by emphasizing women's right to individualized and alternative births" (2005: 261). However, Beckett ends by saying: "Indeed, there is overwhelming evidence that the social organization and practices of independent midwifery are more consistent with women's interest in their own health and well-being, the health and well-being of their babies, and,

more indirectly, all consumers of health care resources that are affected by the injudicious use of those resources. Its existence also generates a body of knowledge that can be used to assess and critique obstetrical knowledge of birthing women; without it, the capacity to do so would be undermined" (2005: 270).

54. I have shown elsewhere how this may lead to the blurring of therapeutic boundaries (Naraindas 2011a, 2011b), and in fact have also argued that blurring may lead to new therapeutic genres or "languages" leading to the creolization of alternative systems such as Ayurveda (Naraindas 2014). But here I am concerned with a cognate possibility: namely, epistemic *contestations* and their ontological *consequences* for protagonists.

References

Alter, Joseph. 1992. *The Wrestler's Body: Identity and Ideology in North India.* Berkeley: University of California Press.

Anaesthesiology Info. 2002. "Anesthesia for Cesarean Section." Available at http://anesthesiologyinfo.com/articles/10032002b.php. Accessed 20 December 2010.

Appadurai, Arjun. 2010. "How Histories Make Geographies: Circulation and Context in a Global Perspective." *Transcultural Studies* 1: 4–13.

Atiba, E. O, A. J. Adeghe, P. J. Murphz, J. E. Felminghtan, and G. I. Scott. 1993. "Patients' Expectations and Caesarean Section Rate." *The Lancet* 341(8839): 246.

Beckett, Katherine. 2005. "Choosing Cesarean: Feminism and the Politics of Childbirth in the United States." *Feminist Theory* 6(3): 251–275.

Bhardwaj, N., J. A. Kukade, S. Patil, and S. Bhardwaj, 1995. "Randomised Controlled Trial on Modified Squatting Position of Delivery." *Indian Journal of Maternal and Child Health* 6(2): 33–39.

Bhasin, S. K., O. P. Rajoura, A. K. Sharma, M. Metha, N. Gupta, S. Kumar, and I. D. Joshi 2007. "A High Prevalence of Caesarean Section Rate in East Delhi." *Indian Journal of Community Medicine* 32(3): 222–224.

Biesele, Megan. 1997. "An Ideal of Unassisted Birth: Hunting, Healing, and Transformation among the Kalahari Ju/'hoansi." In *Childbirth and Authoritative Knowledge: Cross-cultural Perspectives,* ed. R. E. Davis-Floyd and C. F. Sargent. Berkeley: University of California Press, 474–492.

Birthing Centers and Hospital Maternity Services. Available at http://kids health.org/parent/system/doctor/birth_centers_hospitals.html. Accessed 18 April 2013.

Butter, Irene. H., and J. Kay Bonnie. 1988. "State Laws and the Practice of Lay Midwifery." *American Journal of Public Health* 78(9): 1161–1169.

Dabner, Jack Duane. 1984. *The Silent Scream.* United States: American Portrait Films. Available at http://www.silentscream.org/. Accessed 8 April 2013.

Davis-Floyd, Robbie E. 1990. "The Role of Obstetrical Rituals in the Resolution of Cultural Anomaly." *Social Science & Medicine* 31(2): 175–189.

Davis-Floyd, Robbie E., and Carolyn F. Sargent. 1997. *Childbirth and Authoritative Knowledge: Cross-cultural Perspectives.* Berkeley: University of California Press.

De Vries, Raymond, Trudo Lemmens, and Charles Bosk. 2008. "The Subjectivity of Objectivity: The Social, Cultural and Political Shaping of Evidence-Based Medicine." In *The Brave New World of Health,* ed. B. Bennett, T. Carney, and I. Karpin. Sydney: Federation Press, 128–143. Available at http://papers.ssrn.com/sol3/papers.cfm?abstract_id=1126443. Accessed 31 March 2013.

DiFranco, Joyce T., Amy N. Romano, and Ruth Keen. 2007. "Spontaneous Pushing in Upright or Gravity-Neutral Positions." *Journal of Perinatal Education* 16(3): 35–38.

Durkheim, Emile. 1982. *The Rules of Sociological Method.* New York: Free Press.

England, Angela. 2007. "Questions for Pregnant Women to Ask a Potential Doctor: Finding the Right Care Provider for You and Your Birth." *Yahoo! Contributor Network,* 14 February. Available at http://voices.yahoo.com/questions-pregnant-women-ask-potential-doctor-197521.html. Accessed 27 November 2011.

Foucault, Michel. 1980. "The Politics of Health in the Eighteenth Century." In *Power/Knowledge: Selected Interviews & Other Writings 1972-1977,* ed. C. Gordon, Trans. C. Gordon, L. Marshal, J. Mepham, and K. Sober. New York: Pantheon Books, 166–182.

Goldstein, Joshua. 1998. "Scissors, Surveys, and Psycho-Prophylactics: Prenatal Health Care Campaigns and State Building in China." *Journal of Historical Sociology* 11(2): 153–184.

Gupta, J. K., and C. Nikoderm. 2000. "Maternal Posture in Labor." *European Journal of Obstetrics, Gynecology and Reproductive Biology* 92(2), 273–277.

Hak, Tony. 2004. "The Interactional Form of Professional Dominance." In *Medical Work, Medical Knowledge and Health Care: A Sociology of Health and Illness Reader,* ed. E. Annandale, M. A. Elston, and L. Prior. Oxford, U.K.: Blackwell Publishing, 351–369.

Haq, Ehsanul. 2008. "Place of Childbirth and Infant Mortality in India: A Cultural Interpretation." *Indian Anthropologist* 3(1): 17–32.

Hardin, Garrett. 1968. "Abortion. Or Compulsory Pregnancy?" *Journal of Marriage and Family* (Issue on *Family Planning and Fertility Control*) 30(2): 246–251.

Hull, Edmund C. P., and R. S. Mair. 1878. *The Europeans in India; or Anglo-Indian's Vademecum, with Medical Guide for Anglo-Indians.* London: C. Kegan Paul and Co.

Hunt, Nancy Rose. 1988. "Le Bebe en Brousse: European Women, African Birth Spacing and Colonial Intervention in Breast Feeding in the Belgian Congo." *The International Journal of African Historical Studies* 21(3): 401–432.

Huxley, Aldous 1966. *Aldoux Huxley's Stories, Essays, and Poems.* London: Dent.

Jasen, Patricia. 2002. "Breast Cancer and the Language of Risk, 1750–1950." *Social History of Medicine* 15(1): 17–43.

Jordan, Brigitte. 1983. *Birth in Four Cultures: A Cross-cultural Investigation of Childbirth in Yucatan, Holland, Sweden, and the United States.* Montreal and London: Eden Press.

Kabra, S. G., R. Narayanan, M. Chaturvedi, and P. Anand. 1994. "What is Happening to Caesarean Section Rates?" *The Lancet* 343(8890): 179–180.

Kapur, Manju. 2006. "The Birth of a Baby." In *Birth and Birthgivers: The Power Behind the Shame,* ed. Chawla, Janet. Delhi: Har-Anand Publications, 123–135.

Kay, Bonnie, Irene H. Butter, Deborah Chang, and Kathreen Houlihan. 1988. "Women's Health and Social Change: The Case of Lay Midwives." *International Journal of Health Services* 18(2): 223–236.

Lazarus, Ellen. 1994. "What do Women Want?: Issues of Choice, Control and Class in Pregnancy and Childbirth." *Medical Anthropology Quarterly* 8(1): 25–46.

Leslie, Charles. 1992. "Interpretations of Illness: Syncretism in Modern Ayurveda." In *Paths to Asian Medical Knowledge,* ed. Charles M. Leslie and Allan Young. London: University of California Press, 177–209.

Loytved, Christine. 2012. *Qualitätsbericht 2010.* Außerklinische Geburtshilfe in Deutschland. Im Auftrag der Gesellschaft für Qualität in der außerklinischen Geburtshilfe e.V. Zwickau: Verlag Wissenschaftliche Skripten.

MacKinnon, Karen, and Marjorie McIntyre. 2006. "From Braxton Hicks to Preterm Labour: The Constitution of Risk in Pregnancy." *Canadian Journal of Nursing Research* 38(2): 56–72.

Mathews, Z., J. Ramakrishna, S. Mahendra, A. Kilaru, and S. Ganapathy. 2005. "Birth Rights and Rituals in Rural South India: Care Seeking in the Intrapartum Period." *Journal of Biosocial Science* 37: 385–411.

Medical News Today, Nursing/Midwifery News. 2008. "Pennsylvania Court Rules Lay Midwife Can Continue Home Birth Practice." 29 May. Available at http://www.medicalnewstoday.com/releases/109062.php. Accessed 19 June 2008.

Mello e Souza, C. 1994. "C-sections as Ideal Births: The Cultural Constructions of Beneficence and Patient's Rights in Brazil." *Cambridge Quarterly of Health Care Ethics* 3(3): 358–366.

Mishler, Elliot. 2005. "The Struggle between the Voice of Medicine and the Voice of the Lifeworld." In *The Sociology of Health and Illness: Critical Perspectives,* ed. Peter Conrad. New York: Worth Publishers, 319–330.

Mol, Annemarie. 2002. *The Body Multiple: Ontology in Medical Practice.* Durham and London: Duke University Press.

Naraindas, Harish. 1996. "Poisons, Putrescence and the Weather: A Genealogy of the Advent of Tropical Medicine." *Contributions to Indian Sociology* 30(1): 1–35.

———. 1998. "Care, Welfare and Treason: The Advent of Vaccination in the 19th Century." *Contributions to Indian Sociology* (n.s.), 32(1): 67–96.

———. 2003a. "Preparing for the Pox: A Theory of Smallpox in Bengal and Britain." *Asian Journal of Social Sciences* 31(2): 304–339.

———. 2003b. "Crisis, Charisma, and Triage: Extirpating the Pox." *The Indian Economic and Social History Review* 40(4): 425–457.

———. 2006. "Of Spineless Babies and Folic Acid: Evidence and Efficacy in Biomedicine and Ayurvedic Medicine." *Social Science & Medicine* 62(11): 2658–2669.

———. 2007. "Epidemics of Fever: Allopathic Prevention or Alternative Cure. Alternative Therapies for Dengue, Chikungunya and Smallpox." *Journal of Health and Development* 3(1 & 2): 45–56.

———. 2008. "Mainstreaming AYUSH and Ayushing Obstetrics." *Health for the Millions* 34(2 & 3): 33–37.

———. 2009. "A Sacramental Theory of Childbirth in India." In *Childbirth Across Cultures: Ideas and Practices of Pregnancy, Childbirth and the Postpartum* (Volume 5 in the series Science Across Cultures: The History of Non-Western Science), ed. H. Selin and P. K. Stone. Heidelberg, London, New York: Springer Dordecht, 95–106.

———. 2011a. "Of Relics, Body Parts and Laser Beams: The German Heilpraktiker and His Ayurvedic Spa." *Anthropology and Medicine* 18(1): 67–86.

———. 2011b. "Korallen, Chipkarten, medizinischen Informationen und die Jungfrau Maria: Heilpraktiker in Deutschland und die Aneignung der Ayurveda Therapie." *Zeitschrift für Ethnologie* 136: 93–114.

———. 2014. "Nosopolitics. Epistemic Mangling and the Creolization of Contemporary Ayurveda." In *Medical Pluralism and Homeopathy in India and Germany (1810-2010): A Comparison of Practices,* ed. Martin Dinges. *Medizin, Gesellschaft und Geschichte, (MedGG-Beiheft 50), Jahrbuch des Instituts für Geschichte der Medizin der Robert Bosch Stiftung.* Stuttgart: Franz Steiner Verlag, 105–136.

Odent, M. 2001. "New Reasons and New Ways to Study Birth Physiology." *International Journal of Gynecology and Obstetrics* 75: 39–45.

Otoide, V. O., S. M. Ogbonmwan, and F. E. Okonofua,. 2000. "Episiotomy in Nigeria." *International Journal of Gynecology and Obstetrics* 68(1): 13–17.

Padmanabhan, P. 2008. "Integrated Service Delivery in Primary Health Care: The Tamil Nadu Experience." Paper presented at Jawaharlal Nehru University, September 2008.

Pickering, Andrew. 2008. "New Ontologies." In *The Mangle in Practice: Science, Society and Becoming,* ed. Andrew Pickering and Keith Gizik. Durham: Duke University Press, 1–16.

Pigg, Stacy. 1997. "Authority in Translation: Finding, Knowing, Naming and Training 'Traditional Birth Attendants' in Nepal." In *Childbirth and Authoritative Knowledge: Cross-cultural Perspectives,* ed. Robbie E. Davis-Floyd and C. F. Sargent. Berkeley: University of California Press.

QUAG. 2012. "Geburtenzahlen in Deutschland." Available at http://www.quag. de/content/geburtenzahl.htm. Accessed 26 December 2012.

Ram, Kalpana. 2009. "Rural Midwives in South India: The Politics of Bodily Knowledge." In *Childbirth Across Cultures: Ideas and Practices of Pregnancy, Childbirth and the Postpartum* (Volume 5 in the series Science Across Cultures: The History of Non-Western Science), ed. H. Selin and P. K. Stone. Heidelberg, London, New York: Springer Dordecht, 107–122.

Riessman, Catherine. 1993. *Narrative Analysis*. Newbury Park, CA: Sage Publications.

Selvaraj, Alphonse, A. Chitra, and S. Parvathy. 2007. *Episiotomy: Real Need or Ritual?* Poonamalee, Chennai: Institute of Public Health.

Smith, Frederick. 2006. *The Self Possessed: Deity and Spirit Possession in South Asian Literature and Civilization*. Columbia: Columbia University Press.

Spock, Benjamin. 2004. *Dr. Spock's Baby and Child Care: 8th Edition*. New York: Pocket Books.

Sreevidya, S., and B. W. Sathiyasekaran. 2003. "High Caesarean Rates in Madras (India): A Population-based Cross Sectional Study." *BJOG* 110(2): 106–111.

Stone, Pamela K. 2009. "A History of Western Medicine, Labor, and Birth." In *Childbirth Across Cultures: Ideas and Practices of Pregnancy, Childbirth and the Postpartum* (Volume 5 in the series Science Across Cultures: The History of Non-Western Science), ed. H. Selin and P. K. Stone. Heidelberg, London, New York: Springer Dordecht, 41–53.

Timmermann, Carsten. 2011. "Appropriating Risk Factors: The Reception of an American Approach to Chronic Disease in the Two German States, c. 1950–1990." *Social History of Medicine* 25(1): 157–174.

Van Hollen, Cecilia. 2003. *Birth on the Threshold: Childbirth and Modernity in South India*. Berkeley, Los Angeles, and London: University of California Press.

Weiss, Richard. 2009. Recipes for Immortality: Medicine, Religion and Community in South India. Oxford; New York: Oxford University Press.

White, David Gordon. 1996. *The Alchemical Body: Siddha Traditions in Medieval India*. Chicago: University of Chicago Press.

Wirtz, Veronika, Alan Cribb, and Nick Barber. 2006. "Patient–Doctor Decisionmaking about Treatment within the Consultation—A Critical Analysis of Models." *Social Science and Medicine* 62(1): 116–124.

Woolley, Roberts. 1995. "Benefits and Risks of Episiotomy: A Review of the English-Language Literature Since 1980. Part I." *Obstetrical & Gynaecological Survey* 50(11): 806–820.

Zimmerman, Francis. 1987. *The Jungle and the Aroma of Meats: An Ecological Theme in Hindu Medicine*. Berkeley: University of California Press.

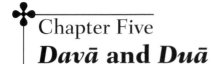

Chapter Five
Davā and *Duā*
Negotiating Psychiatry and Ritual Healing of Madness

Helene Basu

Introduction

Pilgrims approaching the *dargāh* (shrine) of the popular Sufi saint Mira Datar in northern Gujarat are today greeted by posters along the main road showing folded hands, a flame, and images of tablets and a syringe, with the words *davā* and *duā* (medicine and prayer) below in Hindi. The posters announce the presence of psychiatry at a pilgrimage site widely reputed for aiding persons afflicted with madness and negative possession. Following recent government reforms, the shrine has become an experimental site for introducing a new program of mental health care services at the grassroots level. Early in my fieldwork, the coordinators of the psychiatric program organized a meeting with psychiatrists and ritual practitioners (*khadims*)—members of the *dargāh* trust—in the office of the shrine. While the *khadims* generally agreed with the psychiatrists that the free provision of psychotropic medicine to "the poor" was a good thing, they voiced skepticism regarding the overall identification of categories of "mental disease" with "madness" occasioned by possession. "If you suffer from mental illness," a coordinator of the psychiatric project claimed, "you may believe in God or a saint and pray to him for helping you out of trouble. That is fine. But you should also realize that praying alone will not solve your mental problems. In order to get well, you need to understand that you have a mental disease which needs to be treated with medicine." A caretaker of the

162

shrine replied: "That may be so. But if you are controlled by an evil spirit or an enemy making you act like a mad person, medicine might not change your condition. Rather, you will need the intercession of a saint to deal with this trouble. You will have a divine experience. So you may get well even without taking medicine."

Such controversies over psychotropic medicine between actors taking psychiatric and religious positions within the wider field of medical pluralism in India present a particular instance of asymmetrical relationships between psychiatry's power to define "mental disease" and religious institutions' assertions of cosmological conceptions of "madness." Current debates in the field of Indian psychiatry revolve around problems of cross-cultural occurrences of schizophrenia and the influence of culture on both symptoms and treatment outcome (e.g., Cohen et al. 2008; see also Jenkins and Barrett 2004). In South Asia, psychiatric institutions coexist with Hindu temples, Christian churches, and Sufi shrines committed to healing madness and negative possession, thus testifying to an ideology of health widely shared across multiple religious communities of the subcontinent. Although demonic possession generally refers to a range of misfortune, it includes manifestations of madness that share some ground with psychiatry's core concern, i.e., psychosis and the syndrome of "schizophrenia" (Littlewood and Lipsedge 1999).

In this essay, I am concerned with relationships between a medical/psychiatric "system" that takes for granted that schizophrenia is a "natural" disease category, and a religious/healing "system" that assumes that sorcery and possession are common sources of madness. While boundaries between religious and other Indian medical systems such as Ayurveda or Unani are as fluid as the latter's engagements with biomedicine (Nandy 1995; Khare 1996: 844; Halliburton 2009), possession and ritual practices for healing madness are not easily accommodated by biological psychiatry (Bhugra 2001), but rather are contested and often denounced as "unscientific" and "unmodern" (e.g., Sax 2009: 323ff.; see also Basu 2009a). Ideological asymmetries are reinforced by the fact that psychiatry is legitimated and supported by the state while possession healing at shrines is not.

This chapter analyzes findings from a fieldwork project on psychiatry and religion in Western India. It is based on research I conducted in Gujarat at different times between 2008 and 2010 with the assistance of Chitra Khare, a trained psychologist. The project also included the making of an ethnographic film (Basu 2009b). We conducted formal and informal interviews at the shrine of Mira Datar with owners and ritual servants (*khadims*), afflicted pilgrims and their relatives, caretakers, psychiatrists, and the staff of the NGO who organize the consultation sessions. For two months, we attended the daily OPD (Out-Patient Department) held by one of two psychiatrists as part of the "*Davā & Duā*" program. In addition, we spent time in the private clinics each psychiatrist maintains in the district town some twenty kilometers away. We also conducted ethnographic research in the mental hospital in Ahmadabad, which is the main organizer of the project, and which provides the stock of psychotropic medicines to be given out free of charge to pilgrims at the shrine.

Because ethnography rapidly turns into history, it should be borne in mind that my account pertains to an early phase of the project. We witnessed negotiations between psychiatrists and *khadims,* and among the *khadims,* some of whom were highly critical of the project. Since we regularly attended the OPD, some *khadims* as well as some of the pilgrims assumed that we were part of the project and initially refused to talk to us. Psychiatrists and the NGO staff, on the other hand, over time began to disapprove of our talks with people about their experiences with spirits, sorcerers, and the saints. It was feared that anthropological research would not confirm and support the project's aims and that it would instead give equal attention to other voices, turning the shrine into a plural arena. Actors involved in the psychiatric project are used to visitors from Europe and the United States who are engaged in mental health work themselves, and thus share basic professional assumptions. This includes the perception of the *Davā & Duā* program as the "development" of public mental health. As ethnographers, we were gradually caught up in snares emanating from the asymmetries shaping the relationship between psychiatry and ritual healing on a global level, though not necessarily locally.

Institutional spaces such as the psychiatric clinic and the shrine enact the relationship between mind and body, and health and illness, in dissimilar ways. This also implies different notions of the self. Within South Asian anthropology, self- and personhood have been subject to much debate arising from contrasting the "Western," physically bounded and autonomous individual with the "Eastern" "sociocentric," "relational" person or the "dividual" (Marriott 1976; Dumont 1980; Geertz 1983; Strathern 1988). More recent studies of Indian self- and personhood transcend this dichotomy by showing that conceptions of permeable bodies, relationality, and transacting dividuals do not exclude self-awareness and individuality (e.g., Mines 1994; Lamb 2002); conversely, ideals of the autonomous, self-contained individual do not preclude dimensions of interconnectedness among Europeans and Americans (for a more general discussion of the relationship between dividuality and individuality, see also LiPuma 1998).

The concept of a "behavioral environment," coined by Hallowell, provides a starting point to explore what kind of behavior institutions like the shrine and the psychiatric setting "ask for." It focuses on the kind of orientations they provide selves with (Hallowell 1955). Each institutional setting constitutes a cognitive and behavioral environment corresponding to and generating diverse types of ideas, dispositions, and thought styles. It brings into focus culturally inflected orientations for selves acting in the world that account for behavioral differences and experiences of illness on the one hand, and for the definition of illness as well as for cultural norms of normal and abnormal behavior on the other. A shrine healing demonic affliction provides orientations for selves as permeable bodies and minds constituted by transacting coded substances with human and nonhuman actors. The psychiatric clinic established within its premises rests on the Cartesian dualism of body/mind and approaches afflictions of mental illness as biological disturbances of the physical body of individuals, more specifically of the brain; by privileging the administering of psychotropic drugs as the main method of healing, it thereby encourages an orientation to that aspect of the self which Jenkins calls the "pharmaceutical self" (Jenkins 2011: 6).

What happens if the "dominant" institution—the psychiatric clinic—is placed within the "dominated" one—the behavioral environment of the shrine? Institutions of healing such as the shrine and psychiatry reinforce different models of the self and the socially informed body in differently structured spaces and by practices administering distinct types of medicine ("divine" and "psychopharmacological"). How do people respond to this experiment and distinguish between the two? Do people deliberately reject the psychiatric model, or try to bypass, circumvent, or compromise with its suppositions? Does the psychiatric model remain dominant, even when inserted into an arena of ritual healing? And if so, from whose perspective is psychiatry, and from whose perspective is religious healing, perceived as dominant? I shall engage with these questions by looking at the making of madness and mental disease within the ritual arena of healing of the shrine of Mira Datar. Ideological asymmetries between "dominant" psychiatry and "subaltern" ritual healing, I argue, depend on the spatial separation of the two institutions; when assembled in practice, boundaries between dominant and subaltern discourses become blurred in processes which Bruno Latour referred to as "translation" (1991). After introducing the political background of the establishment of the *Davā & Duā* project as a community mental health project, I shall then explore the relationships among the institution of the shrine, Sufi cosmological concepts of madness, and embodied practices of possession healing. The next section will demonstrate that people's decisions to seek health at a shrine, rather than always being self-evident outcomes of the dispositions of the habitus (Bourdieu 1990), may also involve circumventing religious or social norms. I shall then turn to the workings of the psychiatric "clinic" within the premises of the shrine, and the practical efforts made by psychiatrists to replace notions of "madness" with categories of "mental disorder" and to convince pilgrims of the effectiveness of psychotropic medicines. The chapter concludes with a discussion of people's perceptions of psychiatric and religious institutions in terms of bodily practices and the ways in which they produce or accommodate experiences of abjection.

Politics and the *Davā & Duā* Project

In 2002, the Indian Supreme Court launched an order declaring " . . . that mental patients should be sent to doctors and not to religious places such as Temples or Dargāhs" (Agarwal 2004: 512). The order was a response to the infamous Erwadi tragedy,[1] which occurred at a Muslim healing shrine in South India in 2001, and included the statement that "chaining of mentally challenged persons is illegal." Extensive media coverage not only suggested that "traditional faith healing" implies inhuman practices by putting "patients in chains," but also that the poor conditions prevailing in government mental hospitals were in dire need of change (see Basu 2009a; Davar forthcoming). In Gujarat, the Supreme Court order coincided with communal violence, which had reached a climax after a wave of violence was unleashed by Hindutva activists against the Muslim minority in the state (Ghassem-Fachandi 2012).[2] The *Davā & Duā* program was established at the shrine of Mira Datar as an attempt to implement the Supreme Court order locally in a political situation charged with communal tensions.

Although in postcolonial India, mental health care services have become diversified through psychiatric wards attached to general hospitals and private clinics, for people diagnosed with SMD (Severe Mental Disorder), confinement—often lifelong—in a mental hospital of the asylum type introduced during colonial rule is still a likely fate. Postcolonial psychiatry, moreover, is shaped by competing discourses between "biological" and "cultural" approaches (e.g., Jadhav 1995; Raguram et al. 2001; Bhugra and Bhui 2007), by institutional reforms of mental hospitals as well as by de-hospitalization (Jadhav 2001). Since the late 1990s, mental health policies have been visibly influenced by transnational developments, including reports on the global burden of mental illness and recommendations of reform made by the WHO to national governments (WHO report 2001). Psychopharmacology is transforming the field of psychiatry globally (Lakoff 2005; Petryna et al. 2007; Jenkins 2011). As Jadhav and Jain point out, "psychotropic medication has become the essence and embodiment of India's community mental health policy" (2009: 61). Mental health professionals tend to assume that people seeking help at religious sites do so "because they have no other option," as one of the founders of the *Davā & Duā* program said. They thus share what in medical anthropology has been discussed as the "marginalization theses," which posits access to biomedical services and psychotropic drugs as the normative benchmark (Ecks 2005; Ecks and Sax 2005; Ecks and Basu 2009; Quack 2012). Another explanation sought by mental health researchers for patients' seeking help at religious places when afflicted with mental illness refers to belief in spirits and possession (Bose 1997; Padmavati et al. 2005; Dein 2008). Both ideas also form incentives for the organizers of the *Davā & Duā* project set up as a community mental health program, a "scientific" complement to belief and a remedy against marginalization.

The initial incentive for the project, however, was the government decree against "chaining the mentally ill" at religious healing sites and, if people were found to be chained, to close them down. While decrying the use of the chain as an instrument of restraint, civic imagination forgot the harsh techniques of physical control applied to "uncooperative patients" in contemporary mental hospitals of the asylum type.[3] In the public indignation over this form of restraint, the chain came to epitomize what modern ideology interprets as the inhuman treatment of the mad associated with pre-Enlightenment. Images derived from the medicalization of madness in European history, such as explored by Foucault, were projected onto present practices of healing possession-madness in India (Foucault 1971). In the recently emerging discourse of psychiatry the issue of "chaining" accorded psychiatry a new function: controlling religious healing.

In multireligious Gujarat, Hindus constitute the majority (ca. 83 percent) and Muslims the minority (ca. 9 percent). There are at least four pilgrimage centers for the healing of madness resulting from sorcery and possession. Only one of these is dedicated to a Hindu god, namely, Hanuman in his form of Kashtha Bhanjan (Remover of Sorrows) (Basu 2012). Mira Datar is the largest in a network of Muslim pilgrimage shrines dedicated to Sufi saints. A team of mental health professionals visited the temple of Hanuman where ritual healing of possession is embedded in the Swaminarayan variety of Hinduism. According to Dr. X., a psychiatrist employed in a government mental hospital in Gujarat, they did not encounter "patients in chains." There was thus no need for further intervention. The case was different with the Muslim shrine of Mira Datar, where the government psychiatrists called in the police to enforce the new government directive. Dr. X. remembered his first trip to the shrine thus: "When we first went to Mira Datar the faith healers did not allow us to enter. They closed the large wooden door of the *dargāh*. They called men armed with sticks and threatened to fight. So next time we had to come with the police. Inside the shrine we found 90 percent of the people in chains." Dr. X. said he felt obliged to follow the government instructions. If the *khadims* had not resisted their visit, they would not have needed to resort to the police. But as a member of the organizing trust explained later, the owners of the shrine had closed the gate because they feared another attack by Hindus. A small shrine at the margins of the ritual landscape of Mira Datar had already been burned down.

During their second visit the monitoring team discovered that pilgrims were "chained." Although the figure given by Dr. X. might be taken as a gross overstatement, formerly there was indeed a separate space within the shrine where men expected to behave violently were restrained. In one of her early publications Beatrix Pfleiderer described it thus: "Behind the washbasin . . . aggressive and virulent male patients . . . are chained to iron rings, which protrude from the secluding wall" (Pfleiderer 1981: 206).The *khadims* called this corner "madhouse" (*pāgalkhānā*). "At first," Dr. X. continued, "we told the *khadim* that we will have to close down the shrine. But then we realized that they depend on its income, so what would they do?" Thinking of the tense atmosphere at the time in the state ridden with religious violence, he added "and we would have probably faced severe law and order problems."

Initially, the mental health team was only concerned with the legal aspect, the prohibition of restraining "mentally ill persons" with chains. But, as Dr. X. explained, they soon realized that it was not a realistic option to follow the state order and close down a Muslim pilgrimage center as large as that of Mira Datar. The psychiatrists therefore sought to win the trust of the *khadims* and eventually suggested to work out a joint program. If the "madhouse" would be dissolved by returning the men restrained to their families or by sending them to the mental hospital, and the psychiatrists would be entitled to run an outreach program inside the shrine consisting of the distribution of pharmaceutical medication to pilgrims, the ritual routines of the shrine would otherwise be left untouched.

Sayyid A. became a supporter of the project. Rather than seeing "chaining" as indispensible to ritual healing, he welcomed the dissolution of the "madhouse": "I never liked the *'pāgalkhānā'* (madhouse) and I'm glad it is gone now. People used to come and leave their madmen with us. What could we do? Such men could not be left to themselves. So they were kept chained in that part of the *dargāh*. Now we no longer allow families to leave an afflicted relative alone. Somebody must stay with them."

For him, the joint program *Davā & Duā* meant a division of labor: "We had always received some pilgrims who were mentally ill (*mānsik rog*), like those men in the 'madhouse' Even before the clinic started here, we had sent them to a psychiatrist in town." Sayyid A. thought that it would make the *khadims'* tasks easier if psychiatrists gave medicine free of cost to pilgrims in need of it—mediating the "saint's medicine" (*bavā kī davā*) to pilgrims suffering from a different "illness" (*bīmārī*), namely, madness resulting from demonic possession and sorcery attacks. Sayyid A. expected that the relationship between *khadims* and psychiatrists would be one of symmetry. But mental health professionals had another agenda and different expectations. Dr. X. explained them thus:

> The *khadims* treat patients by unknown religious rituals [*sic*] and faith-based methods. The treatment lasts from one day to sixty days or more. These patients are made to stay in the premises of the *dargāh* for long periods of time. When the illness becomes chronic, these patients are also chained and kept tied in the premises of the *dargāh*. This leads to further complications. We felt a very strong need to sensitize the *khadims* that mentally ill patients gain from scientific treatment [with psychoactive medication]. Therefore we had implemented the program of *Davā & Duā*. We want it to become an example of innovative community mental health care. Patients are treated scientifically along with faith-based methods.

The Behavioral Environment of Mira Datar: Madness and Permeable Bodies

The *dargāh* of the Sufi saint Sayyid Ali Mira Datar is situated on the outskirts of a prosperous village in northern Gujarat dominated by landowners of the Hindu Patel caste (for an earlier study of Mira Datar, see Pfleiderer 2006). The owners and *khadims* of the shrine, an extended kinship group of Sayyid, live close by in a neighborhood of approximately 150 households. According to the narratives told by the *khadims*, Mira Datar was a medieval warrior who sacrificed his life in a war against a sorcerer-king. The walled compound of Mira Datar's tomb forms the center within a ritual geography encompassing two larger shrines as well as numerous other tombs belonging to patrilineal ancestors of Mira Datar or his *khadims*. Annually, the number of pilgrims seeking relief from suffering amounts to several thousand; they are or become clients of one of about 600 *khadims*. The clientele of the *khadims* at the Mira Datar complex is cosmopolitan. Pilgrims come from all over Western India, many of them being migrant workers in Gujarat.

So-called Non-Resident-Indians (NRI) living in the U.K. or United States visit the shrine too. In addition to Sunni Muslims, who form the majority of pilgrims, one also encounters Hindus, and occasionally Jains and Sikhs. According to widespread Hindu beliefs, Sufi saints hold great powers against sorcery.

The shrine specializes in countering sorcery and negative possession. Sufism's association with possession, sorcery, black magic, and the exorcism of *jinn* (Islamic spirits) is widespread (Haq 2010). Equally common is the idea that spirit possession and black magic can produce all kinds of misfortune and illnesses including madness.[4] In South Asian Muslim cultures, exorcism is performed by individual healers and diviners (Kakar 1982; Ewing 1984), as well as by Sufi shrines where healing takes the form of a battle between the *pir* or *bavā* (saint) and the forces of evil in the body of the afflicted self (Pirani et al. 2008; Basu 2010a).

As Janice Boddy highlighted in her review of the anthropological literature on possession phenomena, possession refers to relationships between materiality and spirit, violence, power, and corporality in a world shaped by fluid and permeable boundaries between human beings and the environment (1994: 407). This overall indeterminacy opens up possession phenomena for ambiguous evaluations. As is well known, Hindu traditions, on the one hand, distinguish positive from negative, illness-inducing possession according to the possessing agent (deities or demons), and, on the other, attribute ambivalent powers of healing and causing sickness to the same supernatural agent (e.g., the goddess and certain gods) (Osella and Osella 1999; Smith 2006; Sax 2009; Basu 2010b). In Sufi traditions, which do not generally allow for possession by God, positive possession may become manifest in other ways. For example, the Sufi cult of Bava Gor includes periodical possession by the saints of its practitioners during annual celebrations commemorating their death (*urs*) (Basu 2004, 2007).

Mira Datar is part of a network of Muslim pilgrimage sites extending beyond Gujarat and specializing in ritual remedies against madness resulting from black magic and spirit possession. Healing shrines like Makhdum Shah and Bavā Gor in the southern part of the state, and Hussein Tekri in Madhya Pradesh, are linked by clients and pilgrims journeying between them in search of health (Basu 2004, 2008b, 2010a; Bellamy 2011). The saints to whom these shrines are dedicated are collectively known as "masters of the spirits" (*jinnat ka sarkar*), each place providing a slightly different model of affliction and sensual experience of living with, and fighting against, demonic possession.

Practitioners at shrines manage distinct ritual procedures while broadly sharing notions of the person in terms of the Islamic tripartite model of body, mind, and soul (*nafs, aql, ruh*) (Kurin 1984; Werbner 1990). This model generally informs Muslim ideals of health combining physical, mental, emotional, social, and spiritual dimensions. Possession and sorcery disrupt the balanced equilibrium among these dimensions, resulting in various kinds of affliction, of which madness provides a most anguished manifestation. States of madness manifest as fragmentations of the unity of a person's body, mind, and soul whereby one becomes separated from one's relationships with others.

At the shrine of Mira Datar, demonic possession is articulated in terms of sorcery's "unmaking selves" by attacking the brain and the mind. Ethnopsychiatric studies have explored sorcery along with possession as explanatory models of mental illness embedded in Hindu, Buddhist, and Muslim cosmologies (Obeyesekere 1970, 1977; Pfleiderer 1981; Bhattacharya 1986; Callan 2012). The discourse of Mira Datar makes a distinction between sorcery and spirit possession concerning the agent who causes the self to be brought under the control of an alien power. Ancestral ghosts, spirits of the dead (*bhūt-pret*), or *jinn* may enter a human being by seizing a favorable opportunity, or they can be "sent" by a human being, a sorcerer, commanding extraordinary "mind-power" (*manas śakti*); that is, occult knowledge and skills in the techniques of black magic (*kālā jādū*). A sorcerer (astrologer, tantric or fakir) acts on behalf of a client driven by passions of envy, hatred, or revenge, and the intense desire to destroy what is good in or for an Other. The source of the affliction experienced by victims is, in this case, another human being, an "enemy" often belonging to their immediate lifeworld. Possession by an enemy stresses permeable boundaries between human beings' embodied selves but reverses transactions whereby persons are inter-substantially constituted as "dividuals." Performances of black magic aim at the social (or actual) death of a (mad) person by severing them from the web of social relatedness and fragmenting the equilibrium of the unity of mind and body.

Shrines involved in healing afflictions of sorcery and possession, however, are subject to modernist critique. This reflects another kind of asymmetrical relationship, this time between ritual healing and reformist Islam. The Muslim elite and Islamic reformers are especially critical of practices that seem to resemble "Hindu" performances. In her study *Arguing Sainthood,* Katherine Ewing has explored political and ideological negotiations in the field of Sufism pertaining to contestations of "tradition" and "modernity" in Pakistan (1997). Her argument emphasizes ideological competition between Sufi positions that form the "basis for individuals and groups to articulate identities in opposition to others" (1997: 90). Writing on Pakistan, however, Ewing does not address the issue of Sufi practices transcending religious boundaries, which is of great concern to contemporary struggles over what should be "true Islam" in India (e.g., Simpson 2006). Moreover, Ewing's analysis remains focused on ideology and the mind as understood by psychoanalysis and thus is not concerned with the embodied dimensions of Sufi practices. These, however, constitute the core of religious contestations and competition between Sufi institutions within the multireligious environment of Gujarat.

Practices of healing madness involve embodied states of possession ambiguously combining enactments of affliction and therapy. Similar forms of ritual healing have been observed in Hindu settings (Pakaslahti 1998; Sax 2009; Sax and Weinhold 2010). At Sufi shrines, *hājri,* the presence of alien agents taking control of a self, one's mind and body—or, as Bellamy pointed out, a state in which the self has been "displaced" within the body-space—(Bellamy 2011), is of central significance. Shrines differ in regard to the media employed by practitioners. Rituals of possession typically work with music, rhythm, drumming—for example at the shrines of Bava Gor and Makhdum Shah, where drums are used to stimulate *hājri*. But at the shrine of Mira Datar, drumming and music are, with rare exceptions, not used for possession healing. Instead, the human voice is the primary means for inducing the forces of evil to make their appearances. For Sufi practitioners who organize institutionalized ritual healing, music, dancing, and ecstatic experiences constitute markers of status distinctions which become manifest in bodily conduct, in more or less restraint, controlled or abandoned bodily movements, in other words in their hexis. The ambiguity of possession is resolved on the level of human practitioners into status distinctions.

The practices of healing madness institutionalized at the shrine of Mira Datar correspond to the dispositions of a habitus shared across religious affiliation by shaping perceptions of bodies and minds open to direct and indirect influences of others (see also Quack, this volume). About one-third of the 300 to 400 people populating the shrine on an everyday basis suffer from some kind of disturbance of the mind (*magaj, dimāg*) that affects their behavior and their emotions. One's brain may be attacked by black magic performed through cursing, or by accepting food given by a relative which transmits her ill desires, or by a tantric ritual in which one's body was drawn on a map indicating the body organ to be harmed, or by a doll pierced with needles. According to the logic of sorcery, madness is an effect of a perversion of social exchange. As Marriott suggested, the processes that "[go] on *between* actors are the same connected processes of mixing and separation that go on *within* actors" (1976: 109). This holds not only for *making* selves by means of transacting coded substances with other people (e.g., Daniel 1984), but also for *unmaking* selves. Moreover, sorcery's *unmaking* selves operates by introducing a dualism into a unified "body-mind-system" (Sax and Weinhold 2010: 242). In the person attacked, it "separates the heart from the mind," as one *khadim* put it, whereas the sorcerer applies disembodied mind-power to enter into the body-mind-system of the afflicted. Or, we may perceive in sorcery an instance confirming Lambek's claim that the "mind/body problem" is universal (though not necessarily Cartesian), and that this "dualism is at once everywhere transcended in practice yet everywhere present, in some form or other, in thought" (Lambek 1998: 105).

Turning to the shrine of Mira Datar, a homology between the permeability of body-mind-systems and porous spatial boundaries of the *dargāh* is noteworthy. Sufi sainthood expressed in blessings (*barakat*) and miraculous action (*karamat*) is closely associated with material objects (tombs). As Sam Landell Mills has shown, the materiality of Sufi sanctuaries collapses dualities between the seen and the unseen, the living and the dead, the divine and the mundane, the real and the imagined (Mills 1998: 32). The shrine of Mira Datar, moreover, collapses dualities between sacred and profane spaces. Thus, the interior of Mira Datar includes a mausoleum, numerous tombs, a memorial shrine for the sorcerer king, rooms for pilgrims, shops, cupboards and cabins of the *khadims*, a mosque, a pond, latrines and taps, an office, and a tree. These heterogeneous places and objects are connected by associations with sanctity, kinship, exchange, and everyday life; they are distinguished by the activities and behavior they call for. The organizing center of these heterogeneous places is the relationship between the *bavā* embodied in his tomb and the sorcerer king metonymically present through a strand of his hair kept in a shrine opposite the feet, at the back entrance of the *bavā's* tomb. Behind the shrine of the sorcerer king is a burial ground of former *khadims* that links the sacred center with the rooms built into the outer walls of the shrine compound. Here, people controlled by human and nonhuman spirits (those of enemies, sorcerers, and ghosts) afflicting madness stay with their caretakers. Thus, when men step out of the sacred center where they just performed the ritual act of offering rose petals to the saint, their gaze may fall on some of the most mundane aspects of life: towels and clothes hanging on laundry lines in front of pilgrim rooms where women are combing their hair or cutting their children's nails.

The juxtaposition of everyday acts and religious performances in one space seems all the more natural since the shrine is the dwelling place of a "saintly household." The domestic is enhanced by means of ritualization (Bell 1992). Mira Datar or the "son's" tomb is surrounded by those of his "father," "father's brothers," and other men and women of the patrilineage; the "milk mother" who suckled the infant is also there, while his "birth mother" (Rasti Amma) is present in a memorial shrine. The "father's mother," Dadi Ma, is not only resident in a tomb deep down in a cave, but also high up in the "kitchen" of the household marked by a dome: "grandmother's grinding stone" (*cakkī*). Ritual healing space is structured by kinship relationships. As has been observed for other systems, possession and ritual healing are often family-centered (Kakar 1982; Pakaslahti 1998; Sax 2009). The behavioral environment of the shrine stresses this aspect by reinforcing people's orientations to family values shared across religious, ethnic, regional, or caste distinctions.

In a comparison of the cultural logic informing religious healing of Catholic Pentecostals with psychiatry, Thomas Csordas demonstrated how each system starts from a phenomenological analysis of preobjective experiences that are turned into distinct abstractions or cultural objectifications (Csordas 1992). Similar processes of objectification are enacted at the shrine. At the onset of a crisis, people perceive in themselves—or a family member—seemingly odd and alienating thoughts, emotions, and behavior. A person might "talk nonsense," stop eating, withdraw in mute silence, experience sudden and incomprehensible rage, behave violently, neglect bodily care and rules of purity, engage in self-harm, or fail in their studies or at work. Such manifestations of behavior remain preobjective as long as they are not subject to interpretation. When a person is taken to the shrine, the reasons for her behavior are not yet determined. At the shrine, a process of interpretation sets in which is accounted for in the name given to pilgrims: "seekers of answers" (*savāli*). In due course, the perception of disquieting forms of behavior of a person gradually becomes focused upon the agents responsible for it, namely, malevolent human and nonhuman spirits. The latter have taken control of the thoughts, emotions, and actions of a person resulting in her "madness." Mira Datar is a major institution confirming and (re)producing through practices of objectification the association among possession, black magic, and madness as a problem of "body-in-the-mind" and "mind-in-the-body."

The shrine provides a setting that Bruno Latour might compare to a laboratory, where—instead of "natural facts"—"divine facts" are fabricated by means of actions of human and nonhuman actors or "existential forms" (2010). "Divinities" in the sense of Latour are "thought-of-beings" which are not substances but modi operandi (2010: 50) and thus involve agency. As Sax convincingly argued, in order to understand healing in general and possession in particular, it is crucial to decenter agency from its location in the Euro-American individual (Sax 2009: 93ff.). Rather than attempting to make out a single substance or actor as the agent of healing, Sax demonstrates that "healing agency is *always* distributed in networks, among agents that are nonhuman as well as human, individual as well as collective" (2009: 133).

Objectification, acting/enactment, and distributive agency are crucial dimensions of experiencing afflictions of sorcery and possession as well as healing at the shrine of Mira Datar. A further important point noted by Sax is that agency implies patiency (2009: 95). Who works upon whom in this Sufi system? The relationship between Allah as the ultimate source of healing and the saints is one of graded agency, and the latter share in divine power through a gift from God, even while retaining their own agency distinct from His; the *khadims* mediate the agency of saints by performing instrumental actions whereby supplicants become connected to the *bavās* and the female saints. They pray with and for clients, channel their offerings to the tombs, and give them the *bavās' davā* (medicine of the saints) such as oil, water from washing the tomb, and rose petals.

Objectification of the spirits or sorcery illness (*bala kī bimārī*) is arrived at through networks of distributive agency assembling human actions, things (the saint's *davā*), spaces, and nonhuman actors. A first step in the process of objectification is the prayer (*duā*) said by the *khadim* with and for his clients. This action channels the divining power of the saints through words and objects. For the prayer, clients sit alone or in a group around a bowl and face the *khadim*. They are instructed to put their hands into the bowl, which contains figures made of green cloth; these are the horses of the *bavā* asked to carry away spirits and other forces of adversity. While praying, the *khadim* holds a broom made of peacock feathers and red threads in his hands, into which the "complaint" of the client is spoken. One of the threads is later tied to the tomb, the other around the wrist of the client. In this way, a bond is established or reinforced between the saints and the client. The prayer begins by invoking Mira Datar and the other saints and then goes on to request their protection for the client and his family's body, mind, and health. This is followed by a list of disembodied, shadowy beings potentially or actually threatening the client's well-being who are asked to be carried away with the *bavā's* army of horses. The term first mentioned in the prayer is *bala*. The term *bala* is common in Sufi languages of possession, but its meaning may vary in religious usage.[5] In the discourse of Mira Datar, the meaning of *bala* combines physical strength (as needed by a warrior) with mind-power (as acquired by a yogi). As an umbrella term, *bala* transcends distinctions among cosmologies by assembling categories of all kinds of inauspicious supernatural agents from Hindu, Muslim, and Adivasi religions. *Balas* are hybrid, powerful beings, agents of destruction and transmitters of the sender's aggression, hate, and envy. They emerge as the major cultural object of which other spirit beings are specific instances. These are invoked in the following list: illness, black magic (*jādū*), sorcerers (*jādūgar*), jinn (beings created by Allah from fire), *bhūt-pret* (ghosts

177

of the dead), ghosts from the cremation ground (*samśān ka śāyā*), witches (*dakan*), human enemies (*duśman*), and then all those who could become potential enemies: family members, neighbors, or strangers.

Clients afflicted by possession are the "patients" of *balas* who have displaced or colonized their personal agency; in turn, it is both the *balas* and the selves of the pilgrims who become "patients" of the saints. Saints give "orders" (*hukam*) and make "decisions" (*faislā*) communicated in *hājri*, or in dreams. Pilgrims' patiency is expressed in numerous ways: once within the behavioral environment of the shrine, they do not act on the basis of personal intentions or decisions but they say that they obeyed an order given by a saint. One pilgrim has come to the *dargāh* because someone in his family received the order of Mira Datar in a dream; a family has received the order to live from begging; another was sent to the shrine of Bava Gor; in general, people cannot say how long they will stay at the shrine until they receive a decision.

Praying *duā* with a *khadim* initiates a newcomer into the cult of affliction. Similar acts of praying with one's *khadim* form a routine practice throughout the stay of a client at the shrine. The *khadim* also provides his clients with material "saints' medicine' (*bavā kī davā*) such as amulets (*tawhid*), water used for cleaning the tomb (*bavā kī pāni*) to be consumed by the client, oil to rub on his body. In some cases, the saints give the order to an afflicting *bala* to wear a chain and a lock in order to control the spirit. Since the *Davā & Duā* program has been established, however, clients have to provide this item of the saint's medicine themselves.

In the process of objectifying disturbing emotions, thoughts, and behavior, *balas* become metaphorical vehicles for an afflicted self to talk about his or her experiences, or the "body-in-the-mind": "*Balas*," Moinuddin, a young man told us, "make the human body their dwelling place like birds build their nest in a tree. They live within and devour a human body. If one doesn't notice it, one is killed. The *bala* feeds on one's organs, drinks one's blood." Even if one knows oneself or an intimate relative to be under the control of *balas*, one still does not yet know if it is a ghost (*bhūt-pret*) or the spirit of a human enemy who brought a person's body and mind by means of black magic (*kālā jādū*) under his or her control. Answers to the questions, "Who did it?" and "Who are you, troublemaker?"

will be received through *hājri,* the therapeutic state of possession when *balas* are challenged by the saints. *Balas* and saints wrestle for control over the afflicted person, who embodies them both through his possession trances. Throughout the day, people embodying one or more *bala* enact the battle waged between saints and spirits at several sites within the shrine (at the memorial shrine of the sorcerer king and at the foot of Mira Datar's tomb, on the terrace and the dome, "grandmother's grinding stone").

The power of the saint's *davā* is revealed in performances of possession healing occurring during and after the evening prayer and the ritual of *loban* (incense). Acts of praying structure the temporal routine of the shrine; *loban,* the morning and evening rites of purifying spaces and people with fumes of incense after a *khadim* has publicly recited a *duā* from the Quran, mark key occasions for the saints to "call the *balas*" to come into the open. Normally, no drums are used in this ritual,[6] the only medium employed is the human voice. After the prayer, a cacophony of screams and shouts fills the shrine compound. All around, people enact their *balas,* near the rooms, around the tomb, in the courtyard, at grandmother's grinding stone. The one place exempt from enacting *hājri* is the mosque. The orderly positioning of women to the left and men to the right of Mira Datar's tomb observed at the time of praying is completely dissolved. Men roll on the floor on the women's side, women sway their bodies in the men's part. Everyone crowds around the vessel of *lobanbattī* to inhale as much as possible of this most precious *davā* of the saint. Incense purifies the body from inside and drives hiding spirits into the open. Refusal to inhale *loban* is a sure sign of a resistant spirit. Those who are not possessed stand around, leap aside when a *hājrivale* runs into them, or try to hear what the *bala* and the *bavā* are saying. Spirits hurl insults, saints give orders. The body of the possessed becomes a container for the battle waged between saints and spirits. The spirits' voices are heard begging forgiveness, giving false promises, abusing the saints who in turn impose punishments. *Hājri* is an intense and often wild experience engaging the "body-in-the-mind" and the "mind-in-the-body"—make one run, bang one's head on the floor, cast somersaults, or moan in pain. Most of the afflicted appear to be in great pain, and to be absorbed in their struggles,[7] even if family members are around. Although no drumming accompanies the ritual, the atmosphere becomes charged

179

sensually—sweating and vibrating bodies, the smell of the fumes, the screams and the extraordinary physical performances by those embodying *balas*.

Through performance, *hājri* spirits and saints are produced as "facts" when seen from the perspective offered by Latour. The simultaneous embodied presence of spirits and saints fabricates them as ontologically real and accessible to experience. By assembling the agency of spatial and other material objects with human and non-human actors in healing, the equally distributed agency of sorcery is wrestled from its secret hiding places. Reinforcing the homology between the space of the shrine and the space of the human body, the *dargāh* provides an arena referred to as an "open court" (*khullā darbār*) where bodies are "opened" (*khullā hājri*) to release the forces that fragment the unity of body and mind. Of all possible orifices allowing entry of spirits into the human body, the discourse of sorcery at this shrine privileges the mouth. Thus, the spirits of sorcerers and enemies become objectified not only through their voices but also in material objects. We were often told by *khadims* and pilgrims how razor blades, snakes, or pieces of broken glass bangles were discovered in a patient's vomit. In most cases, an—absent—close relative or a neighbor is suspected or identified as the source of a patient's suffering. Innocent-looking items of food seemingly given "from the heart" turn out to have been encoded with destructive emotions of envy and hatred. By means of techniques of black magic employed in a relationship of exchange, food becomes transformed in a victim's body into the deadly weapons of a secret enemy aiming to crush the object of hatred. This once again confirms the point made by Marriott concerning the homology between processes between and within persons. The well-being of permeable bodies and minds is not a stable condition but is continually under threat from the dark sides of sociality.

Circumventing Dominant Ideologies

It has often been observed in the literature of medical anthropology that patients may circulate among different medical institutions. For example, it has been argued that medical concepts are less crucial for patients' health-seeking behavior than the person of the healer (Kakar 1982; Barrett 2008: 25). As Halliburton demonstrated in his study on health seeking in Kerala, not only the provider of treatment is important but also the aesthetic experiences that patients have within different institutional settings (Halliburton 2009). By regularly returning to a religious place or spending years in it, Halliburton argued, patients found a "way of managing problems of [mental affliction]" (2009: 182). At Mira Datar, too, it is rather common that pilgrims confronting a crisis of madness have sought help at other institutions—religious, biomedical, psychiatric—before settling for the "saints' medicine." Some patients live at the shrine for years.

Among the participants in my research at least, the decision was never made solely by the afflicted person—especially if someone had already received the diagnosis of "schizophrenia." In accordance with the paradigm of sociality, the problem is usually not understood to concern exclusively the afflicted individual but the web of social relationships and the family. Moreover, as the following cases of afflicted persons show, ideologies of health may change and diversify in a particular social setting, while unambiguous definitions of "dominant" concepts become blurred. Decisions to resist or circumvent treatment may also be influenced by asymmetrical relationships of power within the family or by considerations of status and the avoidance of social stigma.

Fatimah and Nasin

Nasin was eighteen years old when we met her. Her mother Fatimah, along with Fatimah's mother, had taken Nasin to the shrine because she had developed some disturbing habits over the last several years. At night, she would pull out large tufts of her once-beautiful thick and long hair, which had become thin and ragged. Fatimah was worried about finding a groom for her daughter. Nasin and her mother lived in a town in Saurashtra; the grandmother stayed with her son in Mumbai. Fatimah and her mother knew the shrine well from previous visits. In the last couple of years, however, Fatimah had not been able to visit the *bavā*. Her husband had died ten years earlier and since then, important changes had taken place in the Muslim Ghanchi caste to which she belonged. Members of the caste council (*paṃcāyat*) were followers of the reformist Tabliqhi Jama'at, which urges fellow Muslims to strictly adhere to Quranic teachings and orthodox practices (Sikand 2001). Visiting Sufi shrines like Mira

Datar was discouraged. According to Fatimah, the local Ghanchi *paṃcāyat* also forbids women to work outside the home. Thus, after her husband's death, Fatimah was no longer able to earn, as she had done before by working as a maid. She and her unmarried daughter had become completely dependent on the son, who was a follower of the Tabliqhi Jama'at and opposed his mother's suggestion to seek help for his sister at the shrine of Mira Datar. Finally, pretending they would travel to Mumbai to visit the grandmother, Fatimah and her mother were able to secretly take Nasin to the shrine. On the first evening during their stay, the saints revealed in Fatimah's *hājri* that Nasin's was a *"bala* problem." Fatimah concluded that either her husband's sister or her husband's brother's wife had carried out black magic against Nasin. "They are jealous of Nasin's beauty," Fatimah said, "because their own daughters are ugly. So they want to destroy Nasin's chances of a good marriage." Although the problem was far from resolved, Fatimah had to ask the *bavā*'s permission to leave after only four days instead of awaiting the saint's order, because she was frightened of her son. What did the son suggest? "He says it's nothing," Fatimah sighed. "'Go to the *moulvi sahib* and pray in the mosque. Things will get right.' But it's not that simple. Nothing will be alright if envious people and the spell of black magic continue to haunt us."

Mumtaz and Aziza

Roughly the same age as Nasin, Aziza had already been staying with her mother Mumtaz in one of the rooms inside the shrine compound for five years. Her mother spoke fluent English. She belonged to a middle-class family of Muslims in Mumbai and said that they were rich. Aziza was sometimes happily smiling, sometimes withdrawn in a sullen mood, and sometimes becoming restless, screaming and threatening to run away. When approached directly, she would smile but never engage in a conversation. "My daughter used to be the best in school," Mumtaz said, "but then someone did black magic against her. Now so many *balas* are troubling her. I have to look after her, that's why we are staying here." Except her husband, nobody in her family knew that Aziza had a *bala* problem and was living with her mother at a shrine. "They think we are abroad," Mumtaz explained. Aziza's *bala* problem was

182

such that she did not "get *hājri*," Mumtaz said, "but I get it on her behalf. The *bavā* tells me what to do with her *balas*." She was always worried that somehow her family in Mumbai might find out about Aziza's condition. At the onset of Aziza's illness, a teacher from her school had suggested sending her to a psychiatrist. The psychiatrist diagnosed "mental retardation"[8] and "schizophrenia" and was about to admit Aziza to a mental hospital. But the husband, as well as Mumtaz, were strongly opposed to this idea. A daughter in the mental hospital would have meant great shame. "My husband told me, 'we can't keep her here. Think of our family and my business. She can't be managed, go and stay with her there [at Mira Datar].'" But staying at a shrine is also shameful. "Many people in our family do not go to shrines. They think it's superstitious," Mumtaz said, "but I know they are wrong." Whether she will ever leave the place depends on the decision of the *bavā*.

Bhakti and Dinesh

Dinesh was about twenty-four years old and, like Aziza, had been staying with his mother, Bhakti, for the past five years in a room within the compound. They belonged to a Hindu caste and came from Mumbai. Dinesh was in the first year of college when he began to develop the strange idea that he was a military commander. He began to attack neighbors and even his father, whom he considered an "enemy soldier." Bhakti told us that Dinesh's father was a successful businessman in Mumbai and that she herself was educated. She was active in the Congress Party until she had to care for Dinesh. The family had initially taken Dinesh to a psychiatrist, she said, who had diagnosed him with "schizophrenia." But the medicine and injections administered by the doctor had had no effect. Dinesh's curious behavior did not change and he could no longer study. Then a friend suggested that Dinesh's father take him to Mira Datar. Initially, Bhakti said, she did not like the idea, as they were Hindus. But her husband had insisted on it, saying that it would not be possible to keep Dinesh at home. Dinesh was "causing too much trouble and embarrassment, our neighbors began to look down on us," Bhakti said. Only briefly did her husband consider admitting Dinesh to a mental hospital, "but that would have been even more shameful. Dinesh in the madhouse!"

183

While staying at the shrine, Bhakti had changed her attitude. "Now I have trust in the *bavā*," she asserted. She also experienced the saints' healing power on her own body. One day, the *bavā's* mother had performed an operation on her during the night. For months she had been worried about something growing inside her; her belly had become huge, but now it had shrunk again. The *bavā* had disclosed to her in a dream that she too was under a spell of sorcery which had attacked her stomach, letting "something poisonous" grow inside her. She was saved by the mystical operation.

Dinesh's trouble, Bhakti said, was a *bala* problem. A Muslim neighbor had employed a sorcerer to strike her son with *balas*. The man was envious (*jalan*), Bhakti asserted, because his own son was not successful in his studies. This the *bavā* had revealed to her in her own *hājri*. Dinesh never experienced *hājri*, as his *balas* were too strong. Still, Bhakti was relieved that since they had been staying at the shrine Dinesh had become calmer, less prone to violence for long stretches of time, and was even able, at times, to talk "normally" with his mother. Although she knew that Dinesh's problem would take a long time to resolve, Bhakti was hoping that sooner or later he would be completely "saved," and that they might receive the order to leave the shrine. Then Dinesh would resume his studies in college.

Each of the cases presented above addresses a situated dominant religious or social ideology bypassed by actors in search of a solution for a behavioral problem or "severe mental disorder" of a junior of a family—and in none was the decision for treatment taken by the patient. Fatimah is faced with a new ideological regime in her caste, emphasizing strict boundaries between "true" and "false" Islam and intruding deeply into her and her daughters' life, both as women and as health seekers. Apart from the religious controversies implied in this modern trend, the dismissal of Sufi practices of healing effectively targets the body and embodied experiences of possession while trying to enforce other technologies of the body and bodily control. This ideology, moreover, cannot help Nasin and Fatimah with their problems.

Aziza's parents circumvented both biomedical paradigms and religious ideologies dominant in an urban metropolitan middle-class environment by preventing her hospitalization. But her case also shows that psychiatric disorders are strongly associated with social stigma. Mumtaz's husband took the decision. His reasons appeared to have less to do with a decision *against* this treatment and *for* ritual healing than with curbing the consequences of social stigmatization. The families' reputation and status can be saved only if Aziza's "madness" is concealed. Aziza, and with her Mumtaz, are excluded from the family, although not completely ostracized. In the social class to which Mumtaz belongs, a "*bala* problem" is as unacceptable as becoming a patient in a mental hospital.

Dinesh's parents, too, bypassed biomedical psychiatry in similar social circumstances and for similar reasons of avoiding social stigmatization. Again it was the husband who made the decision. For Bhakti, moreover, seeking help for her son at a Sufi shrine demanded that she transcend her religious identity as a Hindu. Moreover, Bhakti accepted, as did Mumtaz, exclusion from her social environment in order to save the status of the family. Through embodying *hājri* in place of her son, Bhakti could resolve her own conflict. Thus, pilgrims who do not see themselves as believers at the beginning ultimately discover themselves to be just as transformed by ritual practices engaging the body and the senses as the people in whom the problem was initially located.

Madness resulting in social fragmentation and the unmaking of selves was precisely the effect of sorcery stressed in the discourse of Mira Datar. Using the metaphor of a human body, a *khadim* explained the situation of pilgrims like Aziza and Dinesh: "Black magic drives families apart. Those afflicted with madness are cut off like a rotten limb from the body." When mental illness is at stake, decisions for circumventing or bypassing dominant ideologies are shaped by asymmetrical gender relationships within the family and confounded by pragmatic considerations pertaining to avoidance of social stigmatization. And although Fatimah, Mumtaz, and Bhakti are not the primary patients, they share patiency with their afflicted children by embodying their *bala*s and the battle of the saints in surrogate *hājri*. The logic of distributive agency of healing thus extends to and links directly and indirectly afflicted selves. The "family centeredness" of this ritual practice includes making room for women who become excluded from everyday social life within their own families because of a child afflicted with a stigmatized illness.

The Running of the Project

The "clinic" was modeled on the pattern of an Out-Patient Department as it is run in a mental hospital. Inside the shrine, the consultations were held in the shrine office, a space routinely used for keeping the files and records of the shrine administration. The clinic was run by two psychiatrists from the nearby district town, Dr. P. and Dr. Y., who took turns offering one psychiatric consultation hour per day at the shrine. A couple of young men from the village and the Patidar caste, who had never set foot into the *dargāh* before, were employed by the NGO as assistants. The assistants kept patient files, looked after the supply of medicine, and helped with the organization of the OPD.

By inserting clinical practices into the space of the shrine, the schemata revealing the culture of biological psychiatry, with its notions of the brain as the location of disease, within a conceptually bounded individual person, were fitted into an arena pervaded by perceptions of relationally occasioned disturbances of "bodies-in-minds" and "minds-in-bodies." Psychiatric treatment also works with networks of human and nonhuman agencies, albeit different ones than those mobilized in ritual healing, whereby "diseases of the brain" become as much fabricated as the sorcerers and spirits made in *hājri*. "We are brain doctors" (*magaj ka daktār*), Dr. P. said, "We make people understand that medicines can heal people suffering from brain malfunction." Dr. P. and Dr. Y. used the international standard diagnostic manual ICD-10 to reach a diagnosis. Both perceived the raison d'être of their practicing at the shrine to be turning "patients of *balas*" into "patients of mental disease" by removing ignorance of the "real causes" of their problems. Following an abbreviated version of the standard psychiatric interview, they inquired routinely into the patients' sleep patterns, appetite, hearing of voices, and thoughts. Still, Dr. P. and Dr. Y. frequently reached contradictory diagnoses—Dr. P. tended to diagnose more patients with "schizophrenia," while Dr. Y. found more people affected by "conversion disorder." Such discrepancies in diagnoses, as Littlewood pointed out, seemed to arise just as much as from "poor communication between patient and doctor" as from the tendency to confound diagnostic labels with—in this case—gender stereotyping (1999: 105ff.). Male pilgrims were more often diagnosed with "schizophrenia," women with "conversion disorder." Psychiatric healing works through files in which the name, age, occupation, place of permanent residence, complaints, diagnosis, and name of the *khadim* of each patient is recorded. The most powerful agent in the psychiatrists' network is their *davā,* psychotropic medicine taken from heaps of packets of medicine carried in bags to and from the shrine.

Initially, few patients were willing to go to the clinic. The following interaction between Dr. X. and a potential patient outside the regular OPD illustrates the difficulties in communication psychiatrists faced with clients afflicted by possession. Once, while strolling through the shrine, we approached a young man whom I will call "Abdul," who had just experienced a vigorous state of *hājri* and seemed somewhat exhausted. Dr X. introduced himself as a "doctor of mental illness (*mānsik rog kā dāktar*)" and we asked if we could talk to him as well as record the conversation. He agreed. Abdul was from Rajasthan and had been staying at the shrine for eight months. In response to Dr. X.'s question regarding his problem, he said he had a "*bala* problem" sent by a rival of his father. The latter had employed black magic, which made Abdul and his five brothers sick. They could have died, he said. Abdul and his brothers had seen doctors and taken medicine, but this had not made them feel better. Dr. X. asked if he thought his father's enemy was responsible for these problems. Yes, Abdul replied; the person had used black magic against him (and his brothers) in childhood because he feared that when they grew up they would become rich. The father's enemy had cursed him, Abdul said, "so that I will never in my whole life be able to get ahead. I cannot progress." Abdul talked for some time about his brothers' illnesses, when Dr. X. stopped him by saying: "I'm not interested in your brother; I want to know *your* problem." He then asked about Abdul's sleep pattern, his appetite, his thoughts, and if he was hearing voices that nobody else except him was hearing. Abdul was taken aback and hardly answered. Then Dr. X. came to the point:

> *Dr. X.:* Do you think you might have a mental illness?
> *Abdul:* No, not at all.
> *Dr. X.:* So you are sure that it's an illness of *bala*?
> *Abdul:* Yes.
>
> . . .
>
> *Dr. X.:* When do you think you will fully recover?

Abdul: This is up to the Bavā. We will be granted the decision from him.

. . .

Dr. X.: OK. Do you feel that you need medicine or not?
Abdul.: No, I don't need such things.
Dr. X.: You don't feel that you need medicine?
Abdul: No.
Dr. X.: You will get better by only doing *duā*?
Abdul: Yes.
Dr. X.: Ok.

Dr. X. sighed and said "let's go. He won't cooperate."
"Patient Cooperation" is a core concept in psychiatric discourse. Patients' "compliance" is thought to be crucial for an effective cure with psychotropic medicine as well as, in this context, to the compliance of the *khadims* within the psychiatric project. Thus, because of the small number of clients turning up at the clinic in the beginning, the *Davā & Duā* organizers suspected the *khadims* of obstructing the successful implementation of the project. Slowly, however, the OPD was gaining ground. Sometimes fifteen to twenty people were waiting in the afternoon, at other times only one or two turned up.

Interactions between psychiatrists and pilgrims turned into their patients lasted from five to fifteen minutes and concluded with a diagnosis entered into the file and a bundle of medicine handed over to them. Often, consultations were held in the midst of crowds of onlookers. People curiously observed the psychiatrist and listened to the stories told by those who came to get medicine. In such a situation, Dr. P. examined a man who was about forty years old, Mahesh. Mahesh had come there for the first time and was accompanied by his wife and mother. They were Hindus and lived in a port town in Saurashtra. According to his mother, Mahesh's behavior gave them much trouble: "Since the past four years he has been doing '*bak bak bak*' [continuously talking nonsense]. He keeps running away from home. He does not work. He would not have come here [to the shrine *and* to the clinic], but the *bavā* has given the order [*hukam*] to do so." Mahesh was made to sit in front of the psychiatrist, while his mother and wife remained standing behind him. Dr. P. asked about his work, and Mahesh said he worked in the port loading and unloading ships. He had difficulties in understanding the psychiatrists' questions but managed to say that sometimes he got "mental" (*mānsik*), by which he meant that "thoughts stayed in his head," that he worried a lot and often could not sleep.

Dr. P. entered "disorganized thinking" as the symptom, "schizophrenia" as the diagnosis, and the name of the medicine prescribed (Haloperidol) into the file. He then told an assistant to fetch the medicines and said to Mahesh: "Take this medicine, you will get good sleep, and the thoughts will also leave you alone. You will get well." The assistant prepared a bundle of tablets and explained to the mother how many times during the day she had to administer them to her son. Dr. P. told Mahesh: "Take the medicine, everything will get well. Weren't you ever given medicine?" Yes, he was, the wife replied, but it hadn't helped. Dr. P. inquired about the doctor they had seen before (a general practitioner) but did not ask about the medicine, assuming that they would not know its name. "Now this medicine will help," Dr. P. reassured them. Since Mahesh was a short-term pilgrim and soon afterward left, we never found out whether Dr. P.'s prognosis was accurate.

At times, psychiatrists seemed to stage their role as distributors of psychotropic medicines almost in competition with the saint's healing. This included the occasional appropriation of the discourse of *bala*. A young Hindu woman from Maharashtra, Vidya, came to Dr. P.'s OPD for the second time. Vidya had been staying there with her mother for six months when their *khadim* sent Vidya to the clinic. Vidya was diagnosed with schizophrenia. Dr. P. addressed her by her name and asked about her condition. She said she was feeling good but could not sleep. Dr. P. then asked if she had "disturbing thoughts," to which she replied that her thoughts were troubled by the *bala* threatening to kill her. To this Dr. P. replied: "But the *bala* problem has diminished now [since you have been taking medicine]. Hasn't it?"

Vidya: Yes.
Dr. P.: Is the *bala* slowly dying with these medicines?
Vidya: Yes.
Dr. P.: Keep taking the medicines.
Vidya: Yes.
Dr. P.: OK? Then the *bala* will be destroyed inside.

Diagnosing Vidya with "conversion disorder," Dr. P. tried to adopt the language of the shrine in order to make his medical intervention seem convincing.

Some pilgrims declined to visit the clinic. Mumtaz sometimes came to watch what was happening in the clinic, but she never sent Aziza. "If she took medicine," Mumtaz said, "the *bala* inside her body would merely get suppressed, and then grow unnoticed, even stronger and more dangerous." Neither did Bhakti take Dinesh to the clinic, at least not in the first few months. Both said that they had not received an order from the saint to give medicine to them.

Whether people reject psychiatric treatment with medicine, such as Mumtaz and Bhakti, or whether they accept it, like Mahesh's or Vidya's mothers, it was always the agency of the saints that people gave as an explanation for their decision. Not even psychiatrists could always withstand the power of the discourse in the behavioral environment of the shrine—even if they alluded to it ironically. While Halliburton discerned the wider influence of psychiatric discourses on possession in the substitution of "ghosts" by "tension" (Halliburton 2005), in the setting considered here "mental illness" did not become a substitute for "possession illness" (*bala kī bimārī*).

Conclusion

Through the *Davā & Duā* program, mental health professionals somewhat uneasily negotiated among attempts to politically control (Muslim) practices of ritual healing, their understanding of mental disease according to biological psychiatry as the dominant ideology of health promoted by the state, and influences of cultural psychiatry (respecting belief). The introduction of a psychiatric clinic into the ritual healing space of a Sufi *dargāh* was envisioned by its organizers as a way to educate "faith healers" and enable them to identify symptoms of true "mental disease." The institutional "loops" of the behavioral environment of the shrine turned out—so far at least—to be stronger. At the most, people have become more conscious of psychiatric categorizations but reject the reduction of sorcery and possession illnesses to symptoms of a *mānsik rog* (mental illness). The psychiatric model has remained relatively subordinated to the discourse of sorcery and possession. Even if some pilgrims agreed to take the psychiatrists' medicine, their acceptance remained dependent on the agency of the saints. The fact that psychiatrists could run a clinic within the shrine premises was conceived of according to the same logic of agency in terms of obeying an order (*hukam, faislā*) from the saint by which pilgrims perceive their own help-seeking actions. Psychiatrists operate a clinic because the saints had "called" the psychiatrists. As shown above, people who are willing to take the psychiatrists' medicine do so on condition that they have received an "order" from a saint or their *khadim*. Acceptance of psychiatric treatment is, however, limited to the confines of the behavioral environment of the shrine. When, as sometimes occurred, the psychiatrist suggested admitting somebody to the mental hospital, people commonly acted evasively and never showed up again.

Psychiatrists may assume that people seek help at a shrine for "mental illnesses" because they follow (false) beliefs. However, "belief" in the effectiveness of the cure is often the result of staying at the shrine and performing behavior which this environment calls for, rather than preceding it. This was illustrated by Bhakti's case. She was unfamiliar with "Muslim ways" and claimed not to believe in them before coming to the shrine; yet she was able to have embodied experiences through *hājri* so that she now "believes." Like many others, she came to believe in Muslim *bavās* through embodied experiences of *hājri*. *Hājri* is more than "traditional behavior" generated by the dispositions of the habitus. Moreover, different sensual experiences provided by different institutions of healing, as Halliburton emphasized (2009), greatly influence people's decision to seek health at new places. While Halliburton's informants talked about the healing experiences they made in different institutional settings as more or less "pleasurable," my interlocutors stressed power and experiences of the divine. The immediate sensual experience of embodying saints and demonic agents is more often described as painful, but its long-term effect is perceived as empowering.

While the treatment methods differ, manifestations of madness may indeed resemble "Severe Mental Disease" (SMD). Both may result in similar consequences of social stigmatization. A family may experience similar difficulties in coping with an afflicted person's "abnormal" behavior, whether she is possessed or diagnosed with schizophrenia. Often, as the narratives of my interlocutors showed, they feel the threat of loss of social status. In such cases, shrines like Mira Datar provide an alternative to hospitalization in a mental institution. Although the *Davā & Duā* program focused on the distribution of psychotropic medicine outside the mental hospital, most pilgrims tended to associate the project, at least initially, with the closed institution of the mental hospital.[9] For pilgrims, the mental hospital represented the power of the state, since admission is usually done through the police and the court. Those who had prior experiences with treatment in a mental hospital stressed its negative effects. They would describe a relative with metaphors such as "s/he has become like a vegetable," "his face resembled a dead man's," or "s/he got a rash." People also resented its closed structures, where sick persons were incarcerated like prisoners and thus isolated from their families. Such experiences confirmed well-known critiques of the physically, cognitively, and affectively disempowering effects of psychiatric treatment, via institutional structures as well as side effects of psychotropic medicines (cf. the negative attitude of the Malayali ritualists discussed by Sax and Bhaskar in this volume). It seems that institutionalization in a mental hospital is more highly stigmatized than staying permanently at a shrine.

The behavioral environment of the shrine, while confirming and naturalizing orientations of permeable selves and bodies, provided a space to live with, or perhaps overcome, the separation and abjection resulting from madness. In this sense the shrine provided a significant alternative to hospitalization and to the social stigmatization associated with it. According to Dr. X. and other psychiatrists, however, pilgrims suffering from behavioral disorders who stay for a long time at the shrine risk chronification of the disease. But as the psychiatric literature demonstrates, chronification of schizophrenia may or may not be prevented by psychiatric hospitalization and psychotropic medication. Treatment may soften or suppress symptoms, but there is no guarantee that syndromes of schizophrenia can be "healed" like a cold. Conversely, some improvement at least in a "long-stay patient's" condition is indeed reported by family members at the shrine.

Moreover, patients living with schizophrenia often do not experience *hājri* themselves, even though they may have been raised in a setting favoring possession as a disposition of the habitus. Those who do experience it speak of possession as weakening when the presence of *balas* is embodied, but as empowering when the saints take control. For example, a young woman said that after frequent *hājri* she felt as if a "weight has been lifted from my shoulder"; a man said he was "purified" from within, another recalled that he "was freed from pain." Acting and being acted upon in the shrine is thus experienced both as protective and as empowering one's body, mind, and soul. Corresponding to the logic of distributive agency, liberation from the affliction of madness may also be achieved by someone experiencing surrogate possession.

The psychiatric clinic within the shrine thus has not become dominant. This is perhaps related to the permeability of the shrines' spatial arrangements. Collapsing dualities between sacred and profane spaces also opens the shrine to diverse institutionalized practices. In an arena where "saints," "enemies," "spirits," and "sorcerers" are fabricated as objectifications of agencies assembling and disassembling body-mind-systems, psychiatrists and their medicine become linked as additional agents according to a logic of practice rather than the logic of separation or "purification" of modern development (Latour 1991). In other words, the psychiatrist's claim to superior, scientific medicine is qualified outside the institutional structures that confirm and naturalize it. A pilgrim who feels liberated from demonic affliction remains bound to the shrine in the role of a spiritual follower (*murīd*) of the *bavā*. The *Davā & Duā* project aims precisely to instill a similar commitment to psychiatry; that is, it aims to convert pilgrims to the *dargāh* into patients of mental disease and "pharmaceutical selves." So far, it has been unable to achieve this.

Acknowledgments

I wish to thank the editors and anonymous reviewers for their careful reading and helpful comments on earlier versions of the chapter. Special thanks go to the pilgrims, experts, psychiatrists and all those who were willing to engage with this project in Gujarat. Research was made possible by the Cluster of Excellence "Religion and Politics in Pre-modern and Modern Cultures" of the Westfaelische-Wilhelms-Universitaet, Muenster sponsored by Deutsche Forschungsgemeinschaft.

Notes

1. During a fire twenty-six people seeking help at the healing shrine in the village of Erwadi died. Their death was attributed to the fact that they were "chained" to trees and thus could not escape. When the remaining "patients" were "rescued" and brought to the mental hospital in Chennai, more than 100 succumbed to a dysentery epidemic.

2. In 2002, a train car in which *kar sevaks* were returning from a campaign in Ayodhya was allegedly set on fire by Muslims. During the ensuing "Gujarat Pogrom," which lasted several months, more than 1,200 people, mostly Muslims, died and numerous *dargāhs* were destroyed, including two minor ones belonging to Mira Datar. The role played by the state and the police in the organization of the violence continues to occupy the courts.

3. During my research I observed in some mental hospitals that uncooperative patients were locked up naked in an isolation cell, beaten, and pulled by the hair to submit to electroconvulsive treatment or forced into a straitjacket.

4. It hardly needs mentioning that Islamic possession shares family resemblances with possession phenomena reported from cultures across the world. It is by now also commonly known that possession practices are part of many religious traditions. Anthropological research has since long deconstructed pathologizing notions of possession proposed in the 1950s and 1960s (Sax and Weinhold 2010).

5. For example, Kakar translates *bala* used by an individual Sufi healer as "demon" and "jinn" (Kakar 1982: 25). In a study of Sufi healing at the shrine of Hussein Tekri in Madhya Pradesh, Carla Bellamy refers to *bala* as "evil spirit" or "misfortune," but she also points out that this word is rarely used; the most common categories are the Hindu terms *bhūt* and *pret* (Bellamy 2011: 140–141).

6. The last day of Moharram, which in Gujarat is also celebrated by Sunnis, provides the only occasion when drums are played by children during *loban*.

7. Enactments of *hājri* at the time of *loban* at Mira Datar resemble performances of possession at the temple of Balaji described by Sax and Weinhold (2010) and Quack (this volume). They differ in terms of the involvement of relatives in *hājri* enactments of affliction. While Sax and Weinhold stress how the afflicted are encouraged to "act out" their pain, this is rarely to be observed at Mira Datar. Here, afflicted persons appear alone but may be closely observed by relatives from a distance.

8. The term "mental retardation" is still used by psychiatrists as a medical syndrome listed in the ICD-10 (F70-F79) referring to impaired cognitive functioning and deficits in adaptive behaviors. As a substitute, psychiatrists use "learning disability" in some institutions such as at UCL/U.K. (personal conversation with Sushrut Jadhav).

9. The Mental Hospital in Ahmadabad was built in 1863, five years after the first "Lunacy Act" launched by the British colonial government in 1858 (Krishnamurthy et al. 2000: 127). For more than 100 years, the structures of the asylum had remained almost untouched. In the early 2000s, the administration of the Ahmadabad Mental Hospital was the first in Gujarat to put the directives of new mental health policies into practice. The dilapidated barracks, single cells like in a prison, and the walls fencing off the mental hospital from its surroundings were pulled down and replaced by bright, clean, and open concrete buildings.

References

Agarwal, S. P. 2004. *Mental Health. An Indian Perspective 1946-2003*, ed. D. G. o. H. Services and M. o. H. a. F. Welfare. New Delhi: Elsevier.

Basu, Helene. 2004. "Ritual Communication: The Case of the Sidi in Gujarat." In *Lived Islam in South Asia. Adaptation, Accomodation and Conflict*, ed. Imtiaz Ahmad and Helmut Reifeld. Delhi: Social Science Press, 233–253.

———. 2007. "Drumming and Praying: Sidi at the Interface of Spirit Possession and Islam." In *Struggling with History: Islam and Cosmopolitanism in the Western Indian Ocean*, ed. Edward Simpson and Kai Kresse. London: Hurst, 291–321.

———. 2008a. "A Gendered Indian Ocean Site: Mai Mishra, African Spirit Possession and Sidi Women in Gujarat." In *Journeys and Dwellings: Indian Ocean Themes in South Asia*, ed. Helene Basu. Hyderabad: Orient Longman, 227–255.

———. 2008b: "Schmutzige Methoden: Geisteskrank durch Besessenheit und schwarze Magie in Gujarat/Indien." In *Un/Reinheit im Kulturvergleich*, ed. Martin Voehler and Angelika Malinar. Munich: Fink Verlag, 47–66.

———. 2009a. "Contested Practices of Control: Psychiatric and Religious Mental Health Care in India." *Curare* 32: 28–39.

———. 2009b. *Drugs and Prayers*. Ethnographic Film. Münster.

———. 2010a. "Healing Madness through Ritual Trials." In *Histories of Intimacy and Situated Ethnography*, ed. Karen Isakson Leonard, Gyatri Reddy, and Ann Grodzins Gold. Delhi: Manohar, 215–238.

———. 2010b. "Possession." In *Brill's Encyclopedia of Hinduism*, ed. Knut A. Jacobsen, Helene Basu, Angelika Malinar, and Vasudha Naráyanan. Leiden: Brill, 416–426.

———. 2012. "Rational Exorcism: Healing Possession and the Swaminarayan Panth." Paper presented at the European Conference of Modern South Asian Studies, Lissabon, 25–28 July.

Bell, Catherine. 1992. *Ritual Theory, Ritual Practice*. New York: Oxford University Press.

Bellamy, Carla. 2011. *The Powerful Ephemeral*. Berkeley: University of California Press.

Bhattacharya, Deborah. 1986. *Pagalami: Ethnopsychiatric Knowledge in Bengal*. Syracuse: Maxwell School of Citizenship and Public Affairs, Syracuse University.

Bhugra, Dinesh. 2001. "The Colonized Psyche: British Influence on Indian Psychiatry." In *Colonialism and Psychiatry*, ed. Dinesh Bhugra and Roland Littlewood. Delhi: Oxford University Press, 46–76.

Bhugra, Dinesh, and Kamaldeep Bhui. 2007. *Textbook of Cultural Psychiatry*. New York: Cambridge University Press.

Boddy, Janice. 1994. "Spirit Possession Revisited: Beyond Instrumentality." *Annual Review of Anthropology* 23: 407–434.

Bose, Ruma. 1997. "Psychiatry and the Popular Conception of Possession among the Bangladeshis in London." *International Journal of Social Psychiatry* 43: 1–15.

Bourdieu, Pierre. 1989. "Social Space and Symbolic Power." *Sociological Theory* 7: 14–25.

———. 1990. *The Logic of Practice*. Cambridge: Polity Press.

Callan, Alyson. 2012. *Patients and Agents: Mental Illness, Modernity and Islam in Sylhet, Bangladesh*. New York: Berghahn Books.

Cohen, Alex, Vikram Patel, and Oye Gureje. 2008. "Questioning an Axiom: Better Prognosis for Schizophrenia in the Developing World?" *Schizophrenia Bulletin* 34 (2): 299–344.

Csordas, Thomas J. 1990. "Embodiment as a Paradigm for Anthropology." *Ethos* 18: 5–47.

———. 1992. "The Affliction of Martin: Religious, Clinical and Phenomenological Meaning in a Case of Demonic Oppression." In *Ethnopsychiatry: The Cultural Construction of Professional and Folk Psychiatry*, ed. Atwood D. Gaines. Albany: State University of New York Press, 125–170.

Daniel, E. Valentine. 1984. *Fluid Signs: Being a Person the Tamil Way*. Berkeley and Los Angeles: University of California Press.

Davar, Bhargavi. forthcoming. "Justice in Erwadi." In *The Law of Possession: Ritual, Healing, and the Secular State*, ed. Helene Basu and William S. Sax.

Dein, Simon. 2008. "Jinn, Psychiatry and Contested Notions of Misfortune among East London Bangladeshis." *Transcultural Psychiatry* 45: 31–55.

Dumont, Louis. 1980. *Homo Hierarchicus: The Caste System and Its Implication*. Chicago: University of Chicago Press.

Ecks, Stefan. 2005. "Pharmaceutical Citizenship: Antidepressant Marketing and the Promise of Demarginalization in India." *Anthropology & Medicine* 12(3): 239–254.

Ecks, Stefan, and William Sax. 2005. "The Ills of Marginality: New Perspectives on Subaltern Health." *Anthropology & Medicine* 12(3): 199–210.

Ecks, Stefan, and Soumita Basu. 2009. "The Unlicensed Lives of Antidepressants in India: Generic Drugs, Unqualified Practitioners and Floating Prescriptions." *Transcultural Psychiatry* 46: 86–106.

Ewing, Katherine P. 1984. "The Sufi as Saint, Curer and Exorcist in Modern Pakistan." *Contributions to Asian Studies* 18, Leiden: Brill, 106–114.

———. 1997. *Arguing Sainthood. Modernity, Psychoanalysis and Islam*. Durham: Duke University Press.

Foucault, Michel. 1971. *Madness and Civilization*. London: Tavistock.

Geertz, Clifford. 1983. "Person, Zeit und Umgangsformen auf Bali." In *Dichte Beschreibung. Beiträge zum Verstehen kultureller Systeme*, ed. Clifford Geertz. Frankfurt: Suhrkamp, 133–201.

Ghassem-Fachandi, Parvis. 2012. *Progrom in Gujarat:Hindu Nationalism and Anti-Muslim Violence in India*. Princeton: Princeton University Press.

Good, Byron. 1994. *Medicine, Rationality, and Experience: An Anthropological Perspective*. Cambridge, U.K.: Cambridge University Press.

Halliburton, M. 2005. "Just some spirits: The Erosion of Spirit Possession and the Rise of 'Tension' in South India". *Medical Anthropology* 24(2): 111–144.

Halliburton, Murphy. 2009. *Mudpacks & Prozac. Experiencing Ayurvedic, Biomedical & Religious Healing*. Walnut Creek, C.A.: Left Coast Press.

Hallowell, A. Irving. 1955. *Culture and Experience*. Philadelphia: University of Pennsylvania Press.

Haq, Syed N. 2010. "Occult Sciences and Medicine." In *The New Cambridge History of Islam*, ed. Michael Cook. Cambridge, U.K.: Cambridge University Press, 640–667.

Jadhav, Sushrut. 1995. "The Ghostbusters of Psychiatry." *The Lancet* 345(8953): 808–810.

———. 2001. "Community Psychiatry and Clinical Anthropology." In *Cultural Psychiatry: Euro-International Perspectives*, ed. A. Tarik Yilmaz, Mitchell G. Weiss, and Anita Riecher-Rössler. Basel: Karger, 141–154.

Jain, Sumeet, and Sushrut Jadhav. 2009. "Pills that Swallow Policy: Clinical Ethnography of a Community Mental Health Program in Northern India." *Transcultural Psychiatry* 46: 60–85.

Jenkins, Janis H. 2011. *Pharmaceutical Self: The Global Shaping of Experience in an Age of Psychopharmacology*. Santa Fe, N.M.: School for Advanced Research Press.

Jenkins, Janis H., and Robert John Barrett, ed. 2004. *Schizophrenia, Culture and Subjectivity*. Cambridge, U.K.: Cambridge University Press.

Kakar, Sudhir. 1982. *Mystics, Shamans & Doctors: A Psychological Inquiry into India and its Healing Traditions*. Delhi: Oxford University Press.

Khare, R. S. 1996. "Dava, Daktar, and Dua: Anthropology of Practiced Medicine in India." *Social Science and Medicine* 43(5): 837–848.

Kleinman, Arthur. 1988. *Rethinking Psychiatry: From Cultural Category to Personal Experience*. New York: Free Press.

Krishnamurthy, K., D. Venugopal, and A. K. Alimchandani. 2000. "Mental Hospitals in India." *Indian Journal of Psychiatry* 42(2): 125–132.

Kurin, Richard. 1984. "Morality, Personhood and the Exemplary Life: Popular Conceptions of Muslims in Paradise." In *Moral Conduct and Authority: The Place of Adab in South Asian Islam*, ed. Barbara Daly Metcalf. Berkeley: University of California Press, 196–220.

Lakoff, Andrew. 2005. *Pharmaceutical Reason: Knowledge and Value in Global Psychiatry*. Cambridge, U.K.: Cambridge University Press.

Lamb, Sarah. 2002. "Love and Aging in Bengali Families." In *Everyday Life in South Asia*, ed. Diane P. Mines and Sarah Lamb. Bloomington: Indiana University Press, 56–68.

Lambek, Michael. 1998. "Body and Mind in Mind, Body and Mind in Body: Some Anthropological Interventions in a Long Conversation." In *Bodies and Persons: Comparative Perspectives from Africa and Melanesia*, ed. Michael Lambek and Andrew Strathern. Cambridge, U.K.: Cambridge University Press, 103–124.

Latour, Bruno. 1991. *We Have Never Been Modern*. Cambridge: Harvard University Press.

———. 2010. *On the Modern Cult of Factish Gods*. Durham: Duke University Press.

LiPuma, Edward. 1998. "Modernity and Forms of Personhood in Melanesia." In *Bodies and Persons: Comparative Perspectives from Africa and Melanesia*, ed. Michael Lambek and Andrew Strathern. Cambridge, U.K.: Cambridge University Press, 53–79.

Littlewood, Roland. 1992. "Psychiatric Diagnosis and Racial Bias: Empirical and Interpretative Approaches." *Social Science Medicine* 34: 141–149.

Littlewood, Roland, and Maurice Lipsedge, eds. 1999. *Aliens and Alienists: Ethnic Minorities and Psychiatry.* New York: Bruner Routledge.

Marriott, McKim. 1976. "Hindu Transactions: Diversity without Dualism." In *Transactional Meaning: Directions in the Anthropology of Exchange and Symbolic Behaviour,* ed. Bruce Kapferer. Philadelphia: Institute for the Study of Human Issues, 109–142.

Mills, S. Landell. 1998. "The Hardware of Sanctity: Anthropomorphic Objects in Bangladeshi Sufism." In *Embodying Charisma: Modernity, Locality and the Performance of Emotion in Sufi Cults,* ed. Pnina Werbner and Helene Basu. London: Routledge, 31–54.

Mines, Mattison. 1994. *Public Faces, Private Voices: Community and Individuality in South India.* Berkeley: University of California Press.

Nandy, Ashis. 1995. *The Savage Freud and Other Essays on Possible and Retrievable Selves.* Princeton: Princeton University Press.

Obeyesekere, Gananath. 1970. "The Idiom of Demonic Possession: A Case Study." *Social Science and Medicine* 4: 97–111.

———. 1977. "The Theory and Practice of Psychological Medicine in Ayurvedic Tradition." *Culture, Medicine and Psychiatry* 1: 155–192.

Osella, Caroline, and Filippo Osella. 1999. "Seepage of Divinised Power through Social, Spiritual and Bodily Boundaries: Some Aspects of Possession in Kerala." *Purushartha* 21: 183–210.

Padmavati, R., R. Thara, and E. Corin. 2005. "A Qualitative Study of Religious Practices by Chronic Mentally Ill and Their Caregivers in South India." *International Journal of Social Psychiatry* 51 (June): 139–149.

Pakaslahti, Antii. 1998. "Family-centered Treatment of Mental Health Problems at the Balaji Temple in Rajasthan." In *Changing Kinship Patterns of Family and Kinship in South Asia,* ed. Asko Parpola and Sirpa Tenhunen Parpola. Helsinki: Studia Orientalia, 129–166.

Petryna, Adriana, Andrew Lakoff, and Arthur Kleinman, eds. 2007. *Global Pharmaceuticals: Ethics, Markets, Practices.* Durham: Duke University Press.

Pfleiderer, Beatrix. 1981. "Mira Datar: The Psychiatry of a Muslim Shrine." In *Ritual and Religion among Muslims in India,* ed. Imtiaz Ahmad. Delhi: Manohar, 195–233.

———. 2006. *The Red Thread: Healing Possession at a Muslim Shrine in North India.* Delhi: Aakar.

Pirani, Farida, Irena Papdopoulos, John Foster, and Gerard Leavey. 2008. "I Will Accept Whatever is Meant for Us. I Wait for That—Day and Night: The Search for Healing at a Muslim Shrine in Pakistan." *Mental Health, Religion & Culture* 11: 375–386.

Quack, Johannes. 2012. "Ignorance and Utilization: Mental Health Care outside the Purview of the Indian State." *Anthropology and Medicine* 19(3): 1–14.

Raguram, R., M. Weiss, H. Keval, and S. Channabasavanna. 2001. "Cultural Dimensions of Clinical Depression in Bangalore, India." *Anthropology & Medicine* 8(1): 31–46.

Raguram, R., A Venkateswaran, J. Ranakrishna, and M. G. Weiss. 2002. "Traditional Community Resources for Mental Health: A Report of Temple Healing from India." *BMJ* 325: 38–40.

Sax, William S. 2009. *God of Justice. Ritual Healing and Social Justice in the Central Himalayas.* New York: Oxford University Press.

Sax, William S., and Jan Weinhold. 2010. "Rituals of Possession." In *Ritual Matters. Dynamic Dimensions in Practice,* ed. Christiane Brosius and Ute Hüsken. London: Routledge, 236–252.

Sikand, Yoginder. 2001. *The Origins and Development of the Tablighi Jama'at.* Hyderabad: Orient Longman.

Simpson, Edward. 2006. *Muslim Society and the Western Indian Ocean: The Seafarers of Kachchh.* London: Routledge.

Smith, Frederick M. 2006. *The Self Possessed: Deity and Spirit Possession in South Asian Literature and Civilization.* New York: Columbia University Press.

Strathern, Marilyn. 1988. *The Gender of the Gift.* Berkeley: University of California Press.

Weiss, Mitchell G. 2001. "Cultural Epidemiology: An Introduction and Overview." *Anthropology & Medicine* 8(1): 5–21.

Werbner, Pnina, ed. 1990. *Person, Myth and Society in South Asian Islam.* Adelaide: Department of Anthropology, University of Adelaide.

✤ Chapter Six
A Healing Practice in Kerala

William S. Sax and
Hari Kumar Bhaskaran Nair

Introduction: Modernization Theory and Health

Although contemporary modernization theory has its roots in Enlightenment ideals of progress, for most social scientists it began with Marx and Weber, both of whom believed that they were seeing unprecedented changes in their respective socioeconomic environments. A central idea for them, as well as for most of those who developed their ideas further, was that modernity was something utterly unprecedented in human history, a new form of human experience brought about by novel forms of industrial production, by the development of scientific rationality, and by the application of technology. Of critical importance for this process was the gradual secularization of society. For Weber, secularization was a function of rationalization,[1] while for Marx, the "opiate of the people" was destined to disappear when the socialist utopia of the future removed the suffering that made it necessary. Such ideas, especially those of Weber, were picked up in the 1950s and '60s by a range of social scientists and historians and developed into modernization theory, which was in many ways the counterpoint to Marxist theory during the Cold War.[2] Modernization theorists believed that the newly liberated, postcolonial states would be guided by social scientific and technical expertise into a golden age of modernity, and that "primordial loyalties" (to ethnic group, regional language, tribe, caste, and above all, religion) would be abandoned in favor of "modern" values privileging secularism, democracy, and science. Government and educational policy could aid this process by clearly segregating science from religion, which henceforth would play little part in public life: indeed, this is a central aspect of what Nehru intended when he advocated the development of a "scientific temper" among modern Indians.

Modernization theory was embraced by the leaders of the new postcolonial states: not only Nehru but also Nasser, Sukarno, and others, who invited (mostly American) academics like Walt Rostow and Edward Shils to become their advisors. The so-called "Third World" was seen by all sides as a crucial battleground between the United States and its allies on the one hand, and the Soviet bloc on the other. Even though they wished to differentiate themselves from their former colonial rulers, these postcolonial states increasingly became recipients of intellectual, scientific, and political programs directed by the "First World" (see Pletsch 1981). "Modernity" was simply too alluring to resist.

But in the end, modernization theory failed spectacularly, for theoretical as well as empirical reasons. On the theoretical side, it was heavily criticized for its teleological assumptions; that is, for the idea that all societies were moving toward an identical form of social and technological organization (represented by Europe and North America, of course). Empirically, it was criticized for the fact that its central predictions never came true. "Democracy" may have become an international buzzword, but it is far from having been universally implemented. Religion has not declined, but rather has grown dramatically in importance. Claims of ethnic diversity have not decreased with the advance of modernization and globalization, but instead have increased (Tambiah 1989).

Why is this important, and what has it to do with "Asymmetrical Conversations"? There are several answers to this question, but perhaps the most important is that, although the "modernization" paradigm has been rejected by many intellectuals, it lives on in certain areas of public policy, and nowhere more so than in the realms of health and development. "Modern," allopathic medicine is bound up, root and branch, with the project of modernization, not only as its vehicle but also as perhaps its most successful exemplar. Despite its undoubted origins in "the West," allopathy has indeed become universal, so that even the most marginal farmer in Ethiopia,

Mongolia, or Papua New Guinea knows what a doctor is and where to find him or her, what an injection is and how to receive it, what a hospital is, and how to comport himself there. Allopathic medicine is the most successful Western export in history: more successful than democracy and capitalism; more successful, even, than soccer. It is now the dominant healing system in virtually every country in the world, and that is why Charles Leslie introduced the term "cosmopolitan medicine" (1976a: 5, 6; cf. Frankenberg 1980: 198).[3] What are the reasons for such dramatic success? Many would say that it is due to its superior efficacy; others point to its long association with colonialism; still others argue that because allopathy is thought of as scientific, it tends to be preferred even when it is demonstrably less effective than home remedies, traditional healing systems, or simply allowing the body to heal itself. Almost certainly the answer has not only to do with its efficacy, but also with the historical circumstances of its diffusion. One of these circumstances is its near-universal association with "modernity," a state that no one can define, but to which everyone seems to aspire. Health-related practices and official health policies therefore provide a useful lens for understanding how modernization theory continues to lead a vibrant existence in the world of public policy, despite what one might call, paraphrasing Mark Twain, the "greatly exaggerated reports of its death." Most state-sponsored health programs (and many nonstate programs as well) are based on ideals and practices that derive more or less directly from modernization theory, including ideals of scientific and technological progress and the efficiency of markets, and practices of centralized regulation and certification of health practitioners. This orientation is part of what Foucault (and many others) have called "biopolitics," that is, "taking the formal principles of a market economy and referring and relating them to, or projecting them on a general art of government" in order to control the population, viewed as a productive resource (2008: 131). More crucially for our purposes, classical modernization theory insists on the strict separation of "scientific" from "nonscientific." Thus, forms of healing labeled "magical," "religious," or "traditional" are ignored or even forbidden by the authorities (see Janes 2001; Sax 2010; Quack and Sax 2010). Much intellectual and bureaucratic labor is expended in order to deny official support to "nonscientific" theories and practices: witness for example the periodic controversies over homeopathy, even in Germany, the land of its birth. In particular, religious and ritual healing is seen as being directly antithetical to modern, scientific practice.[4]

Those policing the boundaries of scientific medicine are called "purifiers" by the historian of science-cum-anthropologist Bruno Latour, who denies that there is, or ever has been, any such thing as "modernity." In his book *We Have Never Been Modern*, he argues that modernity is not a fact but rather an ideology, a way for "the West" to distinguish itself from "the Rest," and for "progressive" people anywhere, West or East, to distinguish themselves from their less-advanced neighbors, in effect saying to them, "We've got it but you don't!" In his humorous yet persuasive style, Latour argues that the ideology of modernity depends fundamentally on the idea that nature and culture can and should be separated, an idea that is paralleled by the distribution of scientific labor between those who study an "objective" and external world using "objective" and external methods (natural scientists) and those who study "culture" (scholars of the humanities). Under this quintessentially modern division of academic labor, those who study the social world are left uncomfortably in the middle, with most social scientists attempting (unsuccessfully) to imitate the methods of the natural sciences. But according to Latour, such a separation is ontologically impossible, philosophically indefensible, and practically unrealizable. Attempts by "purifiers" to enforce the nature/culture separation create "monsters"; that is, phenomena that publicly and obstinately confound the distinction. One of the many examples Latour provides is climate change: is it a natural phenomenon, or a cultural one? The question is absurd, since the mutual entanglements of nature and culture in the causes, course, and consequences of climate change are so great that they cannot be separated. Latour goes on to argue that the ideology of modernity is inherently asymmetrical because it insists on the greater validity and higher value of natural as opposed to social science. This accounts for the professional ambivalence of social scientists, most of whom attempt to glean some of the prestige (and funding!) associated with natural sciences by employing their methods to constitute and analyze social objects "politics," "economics," and "society," but still fail to be recognized as "truly scientific" by the natural scientists at the top of the hierarchy.

All of this plays itself out very clearly in the relationship that is the focus of this article: namely, that between the sciences of the body and those of the mind. Because measurability is widely regarded as one of the most important criteria of scientific authority, and because material objects and processes like bone cells and blood pressure are much more readily weighed and measured than psychological objects like neuroses and psychoses, a ranked division of scientific labor emerges along clearly defined disciplinary lines: the precise, biological sciences of the body are more prestigious (and better funded) than the rather imprecise sciences of the mind.[5] A look around the landscape of the university, or the institutes of health research, or the various health-related therapies on offer in any large town or city, confirms the point with great clarity: the more a discipline is able to materialize its object and employ a quantitative methodology, the higher it rises on the scale of scientific prestige, research funding, and consultation fees. Conversely, the worse it is at measuring and counting, and the more it makes use of concepts like "mind" and "consciousness," the more likely it is to be relegated to the sidelines, to the social sciences, or even (God forbid!) to the arts faculty. This also explains why drug therapies continue to replace talk therapies as the preferred method of psychiatrists, and why there is such a demand in the universities for neuropsychologists rather than, say, phenomenologically oriented psychiatrists.

Cosmopolitan medicine is thought to represent the best current scientific knowledge, unsullied by culture and history, to be the most accurate reflection of the natural world of health and disease "as they really are," whereas alternative medicine or traditional systems like Ayurveda are thought to be sustained by human credibility and wishful thinking—that is, by "culture"—but not by science. The ideology of modernity generates a practically endless series of oppositions out of the fundamental distinction between nature and culture, and these oppositions are invariably asymmetrical, not only between the natural and the social sciences, but also, for example, between drug-based psychiatry and talk-based clinical psychology, or between cosmopolitan medicine (the natural science of health and healing) and religious healing (a non- or even premodern "cultural" activity). According to the modernists, medicine and religion can and must be kept separate; indeed, medicine could become truly scientific only after this separation had been made and enforced. And this anti-religious bias is particularly strong within the discipline of psychiatry, a point that is discussed at length at the end of this chapter.

All of these themes played out in the "modernization" of Ayurveda during the colonial era, a process that continues today. This process may well have involved the "deritualization" of ayurvedic practice; however there is no way of knowing how large a part religion and ritual played in precolonial Ayurvedic practice, since there are practically no empirical descriptions of it. Most *vaidyas* (Ayurvedic physicians) were Hindus and lived in a Hindu environment, so we can assume that religion and ritual played a significant role in their practice as well as their domestic lives. Contemporary anthropologists have documented how *vaidyas* sometimes perform rituals directly related to their practice (Nichter and Nichter 2010), and it seems reasonable to assume that such rituals were more common in the precolonial era. The influential medical historian Leslie argued that over the centuries, the relatively secular and rational medicine of the classical Ayurvedic texts "became more and more saturated with religious and ritual practices, but that in the 19th and 20th centuries this process was reversed by an emergent class of English-educated professionals who revived Ayurveda along rationalist lines, purging it of religious influences" (1976b: 360). Contemporary *vaidyas* are trained in Ayurvedic colleges that, for all intents and purposes, mimic the curricula and pedagogy of allopathic medical schools (Naraindas 2006). The classical language of Sanskrit, which was once fundamental to Ayurvedic education, continues to decline in importance in these schools, traditional anatomy has been completely replaced by Western-style anatomy, and most graduates go on after graduation to practice a kind of inferior allopathy (Langford 2002). In previous eras, many *vaidyas* grew their own medicinal plants, but now such practitioners are nearly extinct. In short, contemporary Indian Ayurveda has come to be thought of as an Indian version of modern, scientific rationality. It has followed the path of modernization by selectively incorporating aspects of science and technology, as well as centralized regimes of training and certification, while at the same time systematically eliminating ritual and religion from its standard practices. For example, Ayurvedic medicines are increasingly manufactured under "modern," industrial conditions, and the rituals previously involved in their production have largely been eliminated.

In what follows, we describe a contemporary Ayurvedic practice that deviates from this modernist norm. One of the authors, Hari Bhaskar, is a professional Ayurvedic physician from Kerala whose

M.A. research constitutes the empirical basis of the chapter, and who spent four months there between July and November 2009. The other, William Sax, is an anthropologist whose numerous publications have focused primarily on the ethnography of the Western Himalayas and on ritual healing. He was Bhaskar's M.A. supervisor, and spent a week with him in the field. The healers described below do not distinguish sharply between science and religion; indeed, they make use of both. They exorcize afflicting beings, but also prescribe modern Ayurvedic medicines. The site of their practice incorporates elements of a medical clinic, but also of a Hindu temple. They maintain the lifestyle of traditional Nambudiri Brahmans (indeed, this is one of the cornerstones of their practice); but at the same time they use internet advertising and participate in a complex system of referrals among medical doctors, Ayurvedic physicians, and astrologers. Is their practice "modern," "premodern," "hybrid," or none of the above? The question is important because it tells us something about how modernity has adapted (or not) to India, how contemporary Indian medical care has adapted (or not) to modernity, and ultimately about whether the distinction between the "modern" and the "nonmodern" is even useful.

The Practice

One enters Poonkudil Mana through a large, arched gateway. The healers proudly say that it "is never closed," symbolizing their openness to the surrounding community and their willingness to treat anyone who walks in through the gate. Such openness is appropriate and even necessary: the healers belong to a high-caste Brahman family living in the Muslim-majority district of Mallapuram in Kerala, and roughly half of their clients are Muslims. The other half consists of Hindus, with a smattering of Christians. The word *mana* denotes a residence and/or family of Nambudiri Brahmins, and this family claims descent from Naranath Bhranthan, a legendary "mad saint" who was adopted and raised by a Brahman family. They claim that their *mana* is architecturally unique, and that the sanctum of the goddess Rakteshvari in the northeast corner was here long before the house was built. The name Rakteshvari literally means "the goddess of blood," and the red-colored *guruti* liquid used during rituals (see below) is offered to her at the end of every day in the central courtyard. But in an interview the senior healer said the family deity was called simply *devī* (a generic term meaning "the goddess") and not Rakteshvari—which might have been an attempt to downplay the goddess's "fierce" nature.

According to a distant relative who was also a *tantri* or temple priest, the healers' powers are partly based on this very house, since they see patients only while sitting or standing inside it, and never perform similar activities outside its premises. He also mentioned the ascetic lifestyle of the healers as an important reason for their success. He said that their healing was successful, not so much because of their medicines, but because they had observed a disciplined and pure lifestyle for centuries, and therefore local people had faith in them. This is perhaps connected to the healers' friendly and gentle manner: they claim to take into consideration everything told by the clients, and to always speak with them as though they were family members. They constantly advised relatives of the mentally ill to speak and behave gently with them. They never used any of the Malayalam words equivalent to "madness," such as *bhranthu* or *Vattu* or *loose* (an English word that is used in the sense of "crazy"). But they also joked about the stigma associated with mental illness. One day while having lunch at the *mana* we mentioned that the food was quite tasty. The wife of the healer who served us the lunch laughed, and said, "Then you must still be ill (i.e. "You must still be crazy"); you've not been cured by coming here." At one level, her joke was a self-criticism of her own cooking, but it also evoked the stigma of mental illness.

There is a bus stop on the busy highway in front of the gate, and patients often get down there, or they take a three-wheeled taxi to the gate, where they enter and walk the thirty meters or so to the large open space in front of the *mana*. They remove their footwear and wait, along with others, to be attended by one of the healers: two brothers and their nephew, the son of a third brother who died in 2005.[6] During our stay in 2009, the healers sat in a small, roofed extension to the *mana*, approximately nine meters square, which was connected to the main house by a passageway (see figure 1). There was a low wall, perhaps 70 cm high, along the perimeter of this extension, with a single gap in it so that people could enter and leave. The healers—all bare-chested and dressed in the traditional loincloth or *mundu* worn by Keralan men—sat on this wall

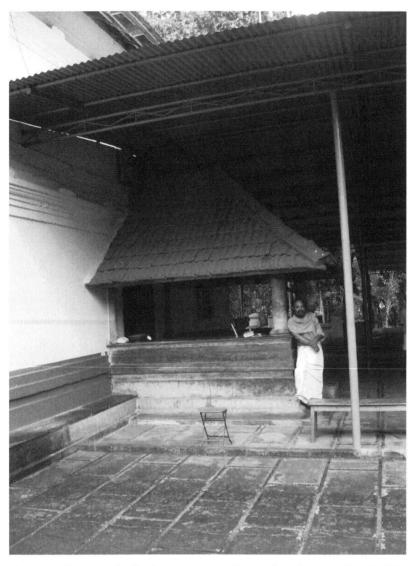

Figure 1. The senior healer leaning against the ritual enclosure at Poonkudil Mana. Photo: William S. Sax, 2009

while consulting with patients. The senior brother often sat in a folding chair that had been placed there for his use. When a patient approached, he or she was likely to see the healers speaking to a few clients or performing their standard ritual (see below), while other patients sat on benches nearby, waiting their turn. The clients were normally subdued and quiet: they did not discuss their problems much with each other, and when their names were called out they approached the covered extension and discussed their problems with the healers, usually in little more than a whisper.

The healers had two main types of therapy: medications and rituals. The medications included a homemade tablet consisting of a paste made of ground herbs and rolled on the palm into a small round pill, which was given for nearly all complaints, from alcoholism to delayed child development. These tablets were said to be charged with mantras, as were other medications produced in the *mana,* e.g., an oil for the head that was made from sesame seeds and herbs, and given to facilitate sound sleep and to "cool the brain." This oil was given not only to those with sleeping problems but also to pregnant women, children with mental/psychological problems, and to those who had already been diagnosed by biomedical doctors and/or psychiatrists as suffering from "mental illness." The healers also dispensed a kind of ghee for internal use, which was prescribed in small doses (e.g., one-half to one teaspoon after lunch and dinner). This ghee, like the oil above, was not only given to prediagnosed cases of mental illness but also given to women for postpartum treatment and to improve the memories of school-going children.

But by far the most popular of the healers' medications was another ghee preparation that they made themselves, which was meant to be used only in small amounts. It was given to almost all clients to smell or taste when they had severe symptoms, or in emergencies. It was used for headache, pain, spasm, dizziness, seizures, and discomforts of varied nature and cause, for immediate external application like a balm, to smell and apply on temple or throat, and to apply on the joints. The recipe is a secret, and we were unable to discover how it is made. It was given in a small plastic vial to virtually everyone who had any signs of discomfort, and they were advised to use it whenever they felt any trouble. The healers claimed that it was ritually empowered, and it was often given together with sacred ash and a thread to tie around the wrist. The clients treated it like a holy substance, smelled it and applied it on their temples, forehead and joints in order to obtain immediate relief. Several clients reported relief from pain, headaches, and similar distress after using it. To the best of our knowledge, no other healer in North Kerala uses anything similar, and there are no reports of such substances by others who have worked on similar healers in the region (e.g., Smith 2006; Tarabout 1999). Already we can see an apparent contrast between the dispensing of "modern" (that is, industrially produced) medications and of homemade, ritually charged ghee. But does this contrast point to a contradiction?

Clients were usually advised to take either *jīrā* water (water boiled with cumin seeds) or cow's milk along with the healers' homemade tablets. The milk used with the tablet had to be from a local cow, and could not be pasteurized milk available from the market. The healers also recommended taking the juices of herbs like *agnimandha* (Skt. *agnimantha*, Premna serratifolia), coconut flowers (Cocos nucifera), and *bhumyamalaki* (Skt. *bhūmyāmalakī*, Phyllanthus niruri) along with the tablets, depending on the patient's complaint. Most clients were also given prescriptions for Ayurvedic preparations like *ariṣṭa* (fermented herbal medicine), or various *gulikā* (handmade pills) available at conventional Ayurvedic pharmacies. The healers also prescribed Ayurvedic capsules and modern, industrially produced tablets with interesting, nontraditional names like *My Mind*, *Perment*, and *Mentat*. These had to be purchased by the clients from specific shops, as most of the conventional Ayurvedic pharmacies did not stock them. One could occasionally see a well-dressed medical representative of one of the companies producing such patented Ayurvedic medicines, carrying his leather bag and waiting in full sleeves and trousers while the healer performed his rituals in traditional dress.

According to the healers, "Western" psychopharmaceuticals were problematic in many ways: they were extremely powerful and dangerous, with unpredictable side effects; they upset the patients' normal balance, resulting for example in uncontrollable trembling; and they had very long courses of use (sometimes lifelong), so that even the allopathic doctors were unsure about when the patients could safely stop using them. Therefore, the healers nearly always sought to wean patients off of them.[7] One method for doing so was to substitute Ayurvedic medicines for Western ones. Those using psychopharmaceutical drugs were advised not to stop them all at once, but to slowly reduce the dose as they improved with the help of the *mana*. Though the healers distanced themselves from allopathic medicines, they maintained a good rapport with the psychiatrists and psychologists in the area, and there were no major quarrels or rivalries. In an interview, the eldest healer mentioned a spectrum of mental conditions, with "schizophrenia" at one end of a scale of severity, and "depression" at the other. But in practice, the language of psychiatry was not used. There were questions about *unmesha*— freshness, clarity, or good feeling of one's mind—but these were part of a series of questions, including those about a blocked feeling in the throat or having tremors.

The healers' practice was not limited to giving medications. They also performed rituals, in particular one called *uzhinjumattal*, to "remove" (the literal meaning of the term) negative energies and afflicting agents from the patients. In nearly all cases, the term used for such agents was *brahmarakshas*, literally a "Brahmin-demon." This is particularly interesting in light of the fact that at least half of the patients were Muslims. According to the main healer, a *brahmarakshas* is a wandering spirit and thus can be removed only by a ritual exorcism that fixes him in an anthropomorphic wooden plank (see our description below). Though some consider the *brahmarakshas* to be a protective spirit, the healers here understand it to be a potent malevolent spirit. They regularly worship it and propitiate it with sweet milk rice. When Sax asked the senior healer if the *brahmarakshas* "really existed" or was just a mental phenomenon, he replied that it "existed for those who believed in it."

The afflicting *brahmarakshas* is never alone, but always accompanied by a number of subordinate demons.[8] In the exorcism ritual, patients entered the covered extension and sat on the floor facing one of the priests, who invoked a local goddess in a burning lamp standing between them, purified the patient by flicking a few drops of water on him or her while chanting mantras, then directed him or her to lift a small brass platter next to an anthropomorphic sandalwood effigy, on which a burning wick had been placed, and to raise and lower it in front of themselves in the typical *āratī* gesture used for "illuminating" deities during worship,[9] thereby invoking the afflicting being who was afflicting the patient. The patient set the platter on the ground, and the priest picked it up and again performed *āratī* with it. Now the wooden image was laid at the base of the lamp and worshiped with mantras, flower petals, rice grains, and water, transferring the afflicting agent into it. Subsequently the subordinate demons were transferred to a burning wick, and from there, into another brass bowl containing water that had been colored red to look like blood.[10] Each step of the process was accompanied by the recitation of mantras, and by offerings of rice grains, water, and flower petals. The client was protected from further influences by the strewing of *bhasma* (ash from previous fire rituals) and rice grains on him or her. At the end of this simple ritual, the priest blessed the patient and directed him or her to stand and rapidly shake his or her hands and feet, thus "shaking off" the last vestiges of the afflicting spirit(s). At the end of each day, the small brass bowl filled with the red water (and presumably also with evil spirits) was tipped into the central courtyard of the healers' *mana*. Was it food for Rakteshwari, the "goddess of blood"?

Although Poonkudil Mana is best known as a center for curing mental disease, Bhaskar discovered during his stay of several months that mental illness was only the fourth most frequent reason for patients' visits. The reported reasons for visits were, in order of frequency:

1. Protection of one's land by performing a ritual to "contain" (*atakkamveppu*) the *brahmarakshas* (see above), a spirit that causes cattle or poultry to sicken and die, or family members to become ill. Hindus as well as Muslims, men as well as women came for this ritual, but most such clients were Muslim men. Some of them presented a record, printed on the *mana's* letterhead and similar to a medical prescription—of similar exorcisms that had been performed there in previous years. They were asked the name of their land, and after they paid ten rupees and twenty-five paisa, their names were written in the healer's diary along with the name of their land. They were then given a sacred thread, some ghee, and ashes to be sprinkled around the house, cattle shed, and chicken coop, the remainder to be kept in a safe place. The ashes and the ghee were to be used on the bodies of those who showed signs of discomfort.

2. Women (mostly Hindu) would visit during the seventh month of pregnancy, to perform a ritual for removing inauspicious

influences, thereby protecting their offspring and ensuring a safe delivery. They were also given medicines after the ritual, following a detailed consultation about their symptoms like nausea, swelling in the feet, pallor, hypertension, diabetes, etc. Once again, rituals as well as medications were used for such clients. The main healer would ask about the hospital and the attending gynecologist, and often showed his familiarity with the patients. Homemade ghee for internal use was given to those who could tolerate it, and homemade oil was given to those with sleep problems. *Mahādhanvantaram gulikā*, a traditional Ayurvedic pill for the health of the fetus, was often prescribed, especially if the client complained of gastric irritation or flatulence. Dietary and lifestyle advice was also given, stressing for example the consumption of leafy vegetables and carrots, and keeping up with household tasks like sweeping.

Lactating mothers also visited the *mana*, usually a few months after birth. Rituals were performed for them while their parents or grandparents held the infant in their arms. It was customary for those who had visited the *mana* during pregnancy to bring the infant after the life-cycle ritual of *annaprāśana* had been performed.[11] Bhaskar also witnessed feeding rituals for older children whose parents had not been able to bring them as infants, and whose later difficulties were then attributed to this failure to visit the *mana* at an early age. Nursing mothers were asked about their supply of breast milk, along with any other difficulties for mother or child. Prescriptions for traditional Ayurvedic medicines like *ariṣṭas* (fermented herbal medicines) and oil for body applications were given as part of the postpartum care for women, and they were also advised to drink cow's milk boiled with the roots of *śatāvarī* (Asparagus racemosus) in case of insufficient breast milk.

3. School-age children and adolescents with learning difficulties from all religious communities visited the *mana* in order to get help. Many had been diagnosed with delayed development while others complained of poor memory, inability to compete in entrance tests, hyperactivity, etc. All received rituals, sacred threads, amulets, ashes, and medicines. The two ghees—one for internal use, the other for external application—and the oil for the head were given to all of them, though other prescriptions

213

varied. In cases of delayed developmental milestones in children, the homemade pill was given with the leaf juice of *agnimandha* (Skt. *agnimantha,* Premna serratifolia) as an adjuvant, while *sarasvatāriṣṭam* (a fermented herbal medicine) was prescribed for those with memory problems. *Sarpandhachurnam* (Skt. *sarpagandhāchūrṇam,* Rauwolfia serpentina root powder) was prescribed for hyperactive children.

4. Patients complaining of mental illness were a very mixed group, belonging to all the major religious communities. Interestingly, most of them had previously been diagnosed and treated by psychiatrists, for example at the Medical College in Kozhikode, or one of the big hospitals in Perinthalmanna. Most had been prescribed allopathic psychopharmaceutical medicines by their psychiatrists, though a small number reported being under the care of, or having undergone counseling with, a clinical psychologist. They were usually accompanied by a close relative, and often carried their medical documents and prescriptions with them. The healers usually asked for "lists," by which they meant their own former prescriptions, medical prescriptions from allopathic doctors, and reference letters from astrologers and other healers, for example *thangal,* Muslim healers. Some clients even presented multiple "lists," for example a psychiatrist's prescription along an astrologer's letter. Once again the actual practice of healers and patients showed a great deal of "mixing" of religious and medical therapies.

   The most important reason for patients shifting the location of their treatment from psychiatrist or hospital to the *mana* was the side effects of psychiatric medicines; for example exhaustion, drowsiness, and lethargy. Some male patients reported that they could not work while taking such medications; others that Western medicines gave only temporary relief from symptoms, whereas the results of the *mana* would be permanent.

5. In addition, there were miscellaneous other problems ranging from skin disorders to liver problems, and from joint pains to an architectural defect in one patient's home, where the toilet had been wrongly placed.

The "indiscriminate" mixture of somatic and religious paradigms could be seen in language used in consultations of healers and clients. For example Amina (a pseudonym), a 28-year-old Muslim girl, was brought to the healer by her father and mother. They had to wait more than an hour, but finally they were called for the meeting with the senior healer.

Case Study 1: Amina

Healer: What is wrong with her?

Father: She is not at all sleeping at night, and not active during the day. She talks very little.

Healer: Yes, there is a slight problem (with her). I will give you a thread and will tell you (what to do with it); we will also do what is needed. Please wait for a little while.

(Amina was very quiet, and the healer did not ask her any questions. He turned to the next client, while the family waited for him to call them again. When he did so, he directed his questions to her.)

Healer: Why are you standing so quietly? Tell me, what is wrong with you?

(Amina remains standing quietly)

Healer: She is not sleeping much?

Mother: No.

Healer: How many days has she been like this?

Mother: It's been a week now.

Healer: Did she take a fright after seeing something?

Father: We don't know.

(Now the healer turns to Amina and tries to make an eye contact with her, but she looks down at the floor. He taps her hand, which is resting on the wooden plank of the half-wall, with the bunch of papers in his hand, to gain her attention. She looks at him, then back toward the floor, but stands attentively.)

Healer: Do you have congestion in the throat, a feeling that something is blocking it?

Amina: Yes.

Healer: Do you have a burning feeling in the belly, which reaches to the chest?

Amina: Yes, sometimes.

Healer: Do you feel a lack of mental freshness and alertness?

Amina: Yes.

Father: She is lying idle in bed most of the time.

215

Healer: Do you have tremors?
Amina: Only sometimes.
Healer: Do you feel a headache, or ringing in your ears?
Amina: I often have a headache.
Healer: Does it get better if you wash your face or take a bath?
Amina: Yes.
Healer: Have you gone to an astrologer?
Mother: We went to a *thangal* (a Muslim priest). He gave her a thread to wear. It did help at first, but later we heard about this place from another relative.

Now the healer invites Amina and her mother to sit on a mat on the floor, and to begin the standard ritual. Once it is completed, the family stands outside and the healer returns to his chair.

Healer: Let her take a tablet in water boiled with cumin seeds, and we'll take another look after a week. Take a coconut, ten rupees and a coin—circle her head with it, and then the heads of everyone in your family, and then around your home and place it at home as an offering. Bring it next time you come here. She should wear this thread. (Speaking to Amina:) You must not take it off! Apply the holy powder to your joints.[12] Do you see the ghee in this small bottle? Smell it, taste it, and apply it to the joints. The *ariṣṭam* (fermented Ayurvedic preparation) that we prescribed should be purchased outside (in an Ayurvedic pharmacy), and should be taken twice daily. The capsules whose names I have written here are also Ayurvedic medicine; you should take two of them at bedtime. They may not be available at a standard Ayurvedic pharmacy, but you can buy them from other Ayurveda shops. She can eat fish, but no meat or eggs. Next time, we will give her ghee, and oil for her head.

These verbal and nonverbal exchanges took about fifteen minutes, although the family had been waiting for over an hour to get an audience, and again for another half an hour before the healer called them forward. There is no real privacy in this practice, and the conversations translated above (and below) occurred in a public space. Interactions between clients were rare and limited, although they could easily see and hear each others' interactions with the healer, if they wished to.

Case Study 2: Lakshmi

One day while Sax was visiting *Poonkudil Mana,* a 27-year-old high-caste (Brahman) Hindu woman came with her mother and elder cousin in an auto rickshaw. It was nearly midday. She got down and approached the healing space unsteadily, chanting Hindu mantras, with her hands joined together in a typical greeting. She behaved as though she were entering a temple. She loudly asked whether this was the temple of *meenkulathi bhagavathi,* a local goddess. With her loud cries and flamboyant manner, she caught the attention of everyone: healers, clients, and anthropologists alike. She drew even with the platform where the senior healer was seated and gazed at him almost reverentially, seemingly confident of his powers. However, he was rather abrupt with her and treated her very much as a doctor would, taking her medical history, etc.

Healer: What is your name?

Client (trembling and looking toward the goddess's sanctum inside the house, still holding her hands still in the worshipping gesture): Please do not pull me, O my goddess of *meenkulathi!*

Healer (loudly and assertively): Tell me, what is your name?

Client: Lakshmi (a pseudonym).

Healer: Do you sleep well at night?

Client: I do sleep at night. But when I was taken to that Nambudiri Brahman to get a protective talisman (*thakit*), I was asked to stay there for three days! I said, "No! What should I do? What does that mean?" Only three days, don't you know what that means? Don't you know? Don't you know?

(She evidently wishes to continue her story, but the healer quiets her abruptly with his next question.)

Healer: What other problems?

Client: I am taking the tablets.

Healer: Oh, so you are taking medicines from a doctor. Why are you taking them?

Client: For mental problems (*manasikamayitulla prasnam*)—but I don't have any mental problems. All of that is gone! But I

cannot stand this pain in my belly—it is blocked, and someone is pulling inside! It is like my goddess of *meenkulathi*,
pulling me (out). It is because someone is doing something
to destroy us.

Healer: Who is doing that?

Client: It is a woman. She was our neighbor. She is doing all this
at the old sacred grove (*pazhaya kavu*). She wants to destroy
us, so that we no longer live there.[13]

(Again the healer cuts her short by interrupting her story.)

Healer: Don't you want this illness to be cured, to regain your
happiness (*sukhamavanam ennille*)?

Client: It will not be cured, even if I visit many doctors.

Healer: Yes, but don't you have the desire to get it cured?

Client: Yes, I do have that desire. But it is not getting better. I will
not allow it to destroy me. I should not be destroyed . . .

*(Once again the healer tries to distract her, as she continues with
what is obviously a story of black magic and cursing.)*

Healer: Do you hear what I am saying? I will do what is needed for
you. You should try to control your mind a little. What will
people say when they see you like this?

Client: They will say that I have a mental problem—that I am mad
(*bhranthanu*)!

Healer: You should not let them say so. You should not give them
such opportunities. Did you eat any food today?

Client (pointing to her cousin): We had lunch at his house. But
the food does not go down my throat. (She starts to weep.)
I want to eat, but the food does not go down! I have such a
desire to eat rice with all the curries, but it does not pass.
Passing urine is also difficult.

Healer: Are you drinking water?

Client: Yes, I drink water, but I pass urine only when heat is
applied. I roll a glass bottle with warm water over my lower
abdomen and it takes a long time. The urine passes only
after one hour.

Healer: Up to which grade did you study?

Client: Twelfth grade: I failed the twelfth-grade examination.
After that I could not go on.

Healer: What was the reason for this illness in the beginning?
What were the difficulties?

Client: Mental difficulties (*manasinu vishamam*).

Healer: What was the reason?

Client: That I don't know.

Healer: Did you ever have a sudden fright?

Client: Yes, once I was afraid seeing a cat.

Healer: When?

Client: It was after I had finished with all my work, at night.

Healer: When was it?

Client: It is not long ago, but I can't tell you exactly.

Healer: How many years have you been taking medicines?

Client: Two years.

Healer: From where?

Client: Dr. X, Dr. Y, Dr. Z. It really started eight years back.

Healer: Do you have tremors?

Client: Not yet.

Healer: Do you sometimes have the feeling of losing control?

Client: Yes, I go to the road and lie down there, thinking that my life should finish. An older woman in the neighborhood came running, a school bus was coming, I knew that. I had done it once before, not knowing that the bus was coming. But this time I knew. I was calling on all the Gods, "Oh my God, oh my Swami, oh Manikadha, help me!" But I don't go to the temple these days. If I go I should offer something there. But it is difficult to go to the temple for marriages because I am like this.

Healer: Did you ever marry?

Client: Yes, I was married once. But he was a peculiar kind of man. At first he was loving, and I told my brother he was a good man. But later it got worse.

Healer: Where was his house?

Client: It was near a large, old Brahman house.

Healer: What was his job?

Client: He was a temple priest (*santhi*). He was a peculiar type, I will not tell about the dirty things, let it go. He is married again now. I have a man I am longing for now.

Healer: First this illness has to get better. If you are like this, then what will people say? So you should get this cured before doing anything else.

Client: I want to lead a normal life with a man.

Healer: Good, but that alone is not enough. You should also control your mind. Who all lives at your home now?

Client: Only my mother and me. My "elder brother" (the cousin who has accompanied her) comes often and gives me money. He is the priest (*santhi*) of a nearby temple.

Healer: Who does all the work at home?

Client: I do. I used to do all the work, but now with this illness I can't do any. My mother has a job, helping the nearby Brahman household. She is blind in one eye. I used to help her, but she is helping me now!

Healer: You should help your mother, and you should control your speech and language. Otherwise people will say something. You should control yourself! I will give you medicines from here.

(The client's mother, who has stayed quiet until now, intervenes when the healer mentions medication:)

Client's mother: She also has a loss of strength in her legs.

Healer: Does she have fever?

Client: No

Client's mother: It is better in the morning.

Healer: I will give you medicines, you must definitely take them.

Client: I have been longing for that man, and . . .

Healer (in an angry tone): Let such things wait! What you must do is get this cured—now! So you should take the medicines!

(The healer takes a call on his mobile phone, confirms his presence, and turns again to the client, who now takes up a new theme.)

Client: Do you know what I wanted to tell you earlier? My father's younger brother came to visit the temple on his sixtieth birthday. He did not bring his wife. He told us that she was sick. We, especially my mother, were afraid of him then. He is a scoundrel!

(The cousin tries to intervene and stop her from talking of such private matters, but she continues.)

Client: I should speak! I will be peaceful only if I speak! I was making bread, and he said, "That is not the way," and showed me how to roll them out. He made two or three, and then came to wipe his hand on me. I shouted, "Don't touch me!" At that time I was engaged. I said, "Don't touch me, a different man should touch me!"

Healer: Let that go, those things are all past.

Client: Then he said, "I am not using underwear these days, I am using only a small loin cloth." Why did he say that to me?" (She starts crying.) Why should he say that to me?

(The healer tries to console her as she weeps.)

Healer: This is because you take it seriously, you should not take it so seriously, let it go.

Client (weeps and repeats): Why should he tell me all that?

Healer: You should ignore such things, they are not so important.

Client: If you say so, I will accept it and be at peace.

Healer: What is your birth sign?

Client: Cancer (*kārttik*).

Healer: You pray there (pointing inside), and I will give you the medicines.

(He looks at the prescription she has brought from a psychiatrist.)

Healer: Are you getting injections now?

Cousin: No, that was before. Now she is taking only tablets. The last tablet she did not take because it was not available in the market.

Healer: Yes, she should continue all of these medicines. (Turning toward the client:) You should control your mind. If you don't do that, you will have thoughts of running away.

Client: Yes, I do have such thoughts: to run away without telling anyone . . .

Healer: You should not do that. You should listen to what your mother and others say. Because although you might think of leaving, you don't know where you would go. When a person like your mother is alone at home you should not do such things.

Client: Yes, my mother also has hearing problems.

Healer: That is what I said. It will be difficult for her if you go away like that. Do you have a blocked feeling in the throat?

Client: No, I don't.

Healer: Do you feel thirsty?

Client: Yes, I did ask for water on the way. But it is difficult to pass urine.

Healer: Do you have problems with your bowels?

Client: Very little.

Mother: It was difficult for her when she was taking the tablets. Then the doctor told her to drink more water.

Client: I eat *kāñji* (rice porridge) now.

Healer: I will give you medicines. Will you take them?

Client: I swear in the name of the goddess (that I will take them). But shall I continue the medicine from Dr. R_____?

Healer: You should also take it. You should not stop those medicines, otherwise your problem will rapidly worsen.

Client: That is why I am still taking them.

Healer: Yes, if you stop them, then you will not know what you are doing. We could slowly reduce them and stop them later. I will do the ritual now. Don't you want it?

Client: Yes, I was afraid seeing the spider, I dropped the vessels.

Healer: Do you take a daily bath? What oil do you apply to your hair?

Client: Yes I took bath today. I use sesame oil.

Healer: I will give you an oil to apply to your head. You should apply it daily and take a bath.

Client: I do have weakness in my legs. That is why I don't take a daily bath.

The healer asked her to wash her legs and face and then enter the *pūmukham,* the space where the rituals are performed. She went to the tap, washed her face, and returned. The healer began the ritual and asked her to pray. She began chanting mantras for the goddess, but the healer told her to be quiet and concentrate in the ritual, which she immediately did. He seemed to have a remarkably calming effect on her. She participated and started to chant, but he told her to keep quiet. During the ritual, when rice and water was flung on her, she looked as though she found it very pleasant. She was given a thread to wear on her wrist, and ashes to put on her forehead. The healer advised her to take one of his homemade tablets morning and evening, along with the juice of *brahmi* (Skt. *brāhmī,* Bacopa monera) and *bhumyamalaki* (Skt. *bhūmyāmalakī,* Phyllanthus niruri) as adjuvants. She was also told to take *drakshādi kaṣāyam* and *mānasamitram gulikā* (an Ayurvedic decoction and a tablet), to be bought from a local pharmacy. She was advised to put oil on her head and to take some ghee after lunch. He told her to take a few containers of his special ghee, which should be smelled, tasted, and smeared over her joints. She should avoid using soap or shampoo on her head. He concluded:

She should certainly be weaned off her allopathic medications. But this should be slow, since stopping them suddenly could increase her symptoms. Usually even the doctors don't know when to stop medications. She should live the life of a family woman: that is our aim.

The woman's cousin paid some money to the healer, even though the latter tried to refuse it. He told the cousin to return in a month and report on the client's progress. She seemed content and, smiling, she joined her hands in respectful farewell and walked back to the waiting rickshaw.

Case Study 3: Madhav

Madhav (a pseudonym) was a 38-year-old Hindu, an engineer from Kerala who had been working in North India for the previous year. He was married, with a seven-year-old son. His family lived in Kerala, and Madhav visited them once every two months or so. His father and a brother were also living in the family home in addition to his wife and son. He had come to Poonkudil Mana with his wife. He consulted the healer and performed the ritual, then sat down to wait for his medications. The healer told us that Madhav might speak Hindi as he was working in the north of India, so that Sax could perhaps talk to him. He asked Madhav to talk to us and to tell us about himself. But Madhav was rather embarrassed; it seemed that although he worked in north India, he could hardly speak Hindi. So the interview was conducted in Malayalam.

> *Madhav:* This is my first time here. I have not yet started these medicines, so I can't say anything about it.
>
> *Bhaskar:* That is fine; we just want to talk to you. What is your problem?
>
> *Madhav:* I get very quickly *depressed* and occasionally *anxious*.[14] I have to first see after taking these medicines, and then only I can say anything about it.
>
> *Bhaskar:* How long have you had this problem?
>
> *Madhav:* Quite a while, but it is there sometimes and it is not there sometimes.
>
> *Bhaskar:* How long has it been like this?
>
> *Madhav:* Quite a while, five or six years. But there are gaps. At times I am *down*; I have *tension*. I have to take these

medicines and see. I have heard that it is good. Do you know? Are they helpful?

Bhaskar: I have also been here only for a month. But there are many people coming here!

Madhav: Should these medicines be taken continuously?

Bhaskar: What did the healers say?

Madhav: Yes, that's what they said. Do you think there is something hereditary in this? My father also is a man of *tension.* I also have too many thoughts. When I have *tension,* I start thinking about the past. But all my thoughts are negative. That is the problem. Anyway, I will take this medicine and see.

Bhaskar: How did you find about this place?

Madhav: I found it on the internet. I looked up sites for depression and anxiety that were related to "herbal" and "Ayurveda," and found it. Then a friend told me that one or two of his relatives had come here and their problems were solved.

Bhaskar: Where does this friend live?

Madhav: In south Kerala, near Thiruvananthapuram.

Madhav returns to the question of the efficacy of the medications, a matter that obviously concerns him, and describes himself as a person who is not suitable for an interview because he has not yet taken the medications. After some time, Bhaskar asks him if he is also here for the mantras and the rituals.

Madhav: No, I came only to have the medications. It was after I had come that I saw the mantras and the rituals. Then I thought, "OK, let's do that, too."

Bhaskar: So you think there is no harm in that. Do you have faith in mantras and rituals?

Madhav: Only *fifty-fifty.* Only that much. At times I have faith, but at times it becomes *fifty-fifty* . . . Yes, sometimes I think, "What is there in it?" When you read the scriptures, you think, "Are they true? Were all these stories realities in the past?" and so on. But then you think, there is a divine power (*śakti*), and the *pūjās* would not be there without this power. There is a *śakti,* but we don't know it, so there is the doubt. But we get a mental benefit. . . .

Bhaskar: How is it now after the ritual? How did you feel?

Madhav: I can take it. One can imagine in one's mind that if there were something wrong, this would have eliminated it.

Madhav received sufficient medicine for two months, and was advised to eat only vegetarian food and then return for a checkup. He hoped that he would be permanently cured by the Ayurvedic medicines. He explained that he suffered from "depression," "anxiety," and "tension," using the English words. He had been under intermittent biomedical treatment for almost seven years. But he made it clear that the duration of this treatment was never more than fifteen or twenty days, because by the time he felt better, he thought that he didn't need the medicines any more. But he found the problems came back because his "self-confidence" and "willpower" was insufficient to provide a permanent solution and help to improve his "self-confidence" and "willpower." But as soon as he was there, he found that the healers also worked with rituals and mantras. Though he had not come to the *mana* to perform rituals, and though he said that he had only a "fifty-fifty" faith in such things, nevertheless he could accept them. Though he related this to worshipping and praying in the temple, he strongly rejected the theory of spirit possession, as well as astrology.

Case Study 4: Ayesha

Ayesha, a 34-year-old Muslim woman, came late in the evening. The main healer was going to the town for some personal matter, and someone was waiting for him. Nevertheless he stopped, asked what are her problems were, and directed her to give her details to Bhaskar.

Healer: What is your difficulty?

Ayesha: My problem is that someone is making me "play" like this. (She danced, turning her hands alternatively to both sides while pirouetting.) Kuttichathan and Chathan Kutti[15] have entered into my body; they are pushing me like this.

Healer: Tell your problems to him (he points to Bhaskar and leaves).

Bhaskar begins to interview Ayesha, and both she and her mother tend to answer his questions simultaneously.

Bhaskar: How did it start?

Mother: I was standing near the well, she was outside and her sister went to the bathroom. Then she cried out, "Mother, my mother . . . something happening to me! I am frightened!"

Ayesha: Someone entered into my body. I cried aloud!

Bhaskar: When was that?

Mother: It was during Ramadan.

Ayesha: After the second day, it was on the third day.

Mother: It was like something had entered her body. But what is she thinking? She thinks that her husband sent (the spirit possessing her). He recently married another girl without her knowledge. And she has three children, three boys.

Ayesha: He had married another woman before me.

Mother (in anger): No need to mention all of that—we were speaking of your present problem! (*To Bhaskar:*) She was with her husband, and what did he do? He brought another woman there! He had built a small house with the money he got from selling Ayesha's gold jewelry. It was thirty sovereigns,[16] and he sold it. He took it all! A woman (in our society) must live with her man, so she did not object. But he gave no consideration for her loss. Even then, she had no major worries, until he brought the other woman to our home.

Ayesha: He kicked me out to bring her there.

Mother: Actually, she was not happy about that marriage. Especially since she was not told about it. Even then she told him, "Please don't make a big drama out of it. Keep her at her own place and give me the money to care for myself and our three children." She was living near his *tharavadu* (family home). But he didn't do as she asked. He had a big, festive marriage ceremony and that made her sad. After all that he broke her spirit completely. He wanted her to stay in the same house where he lived with his new wife: she protested and did not want to go, but he took her there by force. Even though his own mother did not accept his new wife, he acted as though Ayesha had accepted her. Thus she was caught in this sadness. Now she is at our home, and says that she will not meet him anymore, and that he should return her money and assets. She used to be quite active, but since going to the well that day she has this fear, and says that he has sent some spirits to harm her. Occasionally she says, "Will you take care of me here? I am going to my husband. I am going back to my children." We are not asking her to go, or to stay, because at a later point she may think it was wrong that we held her with us.

Ayesha: My children are often calling me to go see them.

Mother: The spirits are making her do strange things. That is why we rushed here quickly.

Bhaskar: How old are her children?

Ayesha: The eldest is fourteen years old, the younger one is eleven.

Mother: She is waiting for her sons to grow up so that they can come and live with her. But she is afraid of her husband, afraid that he will harm her. He didn't even buy a single piece of clothing for her—we did, even at Ramadan! And she was happy, too, laughing and playing. It is only since that one day, at 4 a.m. in the morning, by the well, that she has started having these problems. She fainted, and then she started shaking and striking out with her arms and legs. That's how it started.

Bhaskar: So there was nothing similar before this?

Mother: No.

Ayesha: I never had any mental disease (*manasika rogam*) before now.

Mother: But now her husband is telling everyone that she is mentally ill.

Bhaskar: And is it a mental illness?

Ayesha: No, something has entered my body.

Mother: Yes, she also says that something has entered her. She did not sleep yesterday. And since this morning she has been speaking too much. But even before that she was beating with her hands and legs on her cot.

Ayesha: I have *sarpam* (the snake god), *karimkutty, kuttichathan, chathan kutti,chekutti pappa, oti murthy.*

Mother: She has been saying all these names. She is also saying that she is going back to her children. She asks us if we will look after her properly! It's clear that he sent them. Her liver was swollen so much this afternoon!

Ayesha: When will you put me in chains?[17]

Mother: Dear god, what is wrong with you that we should put you in chains? You should not say such things!

Ayesha: Then how will these beings go out of me?

Bhaskar: The healer will come now, please wait.

Mother: We came here saying, "We are going to the Ayurvedic mental health hospital in Kottakkal." But that medicine is not suitable. She had an episode of *strī-roga* (leukorrhea) when she took that medicine.

Ayesha: I am afraid, I am afraid! Will you leave me now and go?

Mother: No, just keep calm.

Ayesha: My husband died because of my prayers, my husband died, I was praying for his death.

Mother: We used to tell her not to pray, but she was always praying so much.

Ayesha: I have got the result now; I have fallen in the pit that I dug myself, haven't I?

Mother: She is also not eating now, earlier she ate normally.

Ayesha: Can you remove those who are with me?

Bhaskar: How do you know that they are with you? How do you know them?

Ayesha: Don't you know them?

Bhaskar: How do you know them?

Ayesha: They have entered me, entered my body.

Bhaskar: How do you know? Have you seen them?

Ayesha: Yes, I am seeing them now! Don't you see them? This is *karim kutti, kuttichathan, chathan kutti, sarpam.* (She starts slithering on the ground like a snake.)

Ayesha: This is *sarpam* (serpent): Isn't this how it moves?

Bhaskar: Where do you see them?

Ayesha: I am seeing them before my eyes. Who will catch this *sarpam?*

Bhaskar: The healer will come now, please wait.

Ayesha: I will not pray like this again, I am separated from my children.

Bhaskar: Where are her children?

Mother: They are with her husband; they came to see her during the Ramadan holidays. They stayed for five days.

Bhaskar: What do the children say?

Mother: They say that their father has done an injustice.

Ayesha: We made that house together. But he kicked me out—for *her!*

Mother: She was living there and taking care of his grandparents. We told her that if he marries again and can take care of another woman, let him do so. You should not worry.

Ayesha: She was also a poor girl, an orphan. I was thinking we could live together. But he pushed me out. I was even washing her clothes.

Mother: He was trying to prove to his relatives that Ayesha had accepted this marriage.

Ayesha: Will this change?

Mother: Yes, this is not a disease.

Ayesha: Can't you catch those who are with me?

(Ayesha's mother reminds her that she has not slept for three or four days, and that it is this lack of sleep that has made her start talking too much. Before that she just lay in her bed and banged her hands and feet against the side of it. Meanwhile the youngest healer arrives, and Ayesha's mother explains the whole story to him, adding the following:)

Mother: First she took the tablets given by the psychiatrist. Then we took her to the Ayurveda mental hospital in Kottakal, when she took those medicines and her leukorrhea increased. She said that those medicines do not suit her. They brought no relief.

Healer: Don't you want to get well and go and stay with your children?

Ayesha: My illness should be cured. It should not return. I feel like vomiting when I eat. (She looks at the motorbike parked near the gate and asks:) Will he push me down if I get on his motorcycle?

Healer: You cannot even stand here, so what will you do at your husband's place? You can return there only after you get well, right? Could you make a complaint with your own relatives, or with the mosque committee, in such a state? After getting well we will talk about it, and get it resolved.

Ayesha: He is calling me back, but I fear he will kill me.

Healer: Such a thing will not happen. I will perform the ritual.

Ayesha: Something has entered my body . . . you should do it now.

Healer: Is she getting little sleep?

Mother: Yes.

Healer: The less sleep you get, the more such unnecessary thoughts will increase.

Ayesha: Someone has conquered me and is going to kill me.

Healer: What would someone else say if one sees all this?

Ayesha: He will say that I am a mental case.

The healer performed the ritual, and asked Ayesha to pray to God during it. He gave her the standard prescription of homemade pills, oil for her head, an *ariṣṭam* (fermented herbal medicine), and a prescription for a tablet and a capsule to buy from a local Ayurvedic pharmacy.

Alternatively Modern, or Never Modern?

A close relative of the healers told us that up into the 1990s, there were roughly twenty-five inpatients at Poonkudil Mana at any given time, and that they focused on rituals and didn't prescribe pills or other Ayurvedic medications, but only their own ghee. The abandoned "in-patient facility," with holes still visible for the chains with which patients used to be restrained, stood in silent witness to this history. But today, the healers make use of various modern networks and technologies, prescribe industrially produced Ayurvedic medicines, and have eliminated the "in-patient facility." So one might be tempted to say that they are "modernizing." However, religious ritual retains a central place in their practice: as we have shown, exorcisms are performed for nearly all patients, and the lineage goddess, said to have been present in this place long before humans were, is one of the main sources of the healers' power.

In fact, it seemed clear to us that the healers follow both "religious" and "medical" strategies with most patients, so that those who come with purely physical complaints are as likely to receive rituals as medications, and those with religious problems are as likely to receive a prescription as a ritual.[18] This is confusing for Indians who, like Europeans, have clear ideas about how to behave and what to expect in a medical practice as opposed to a temple or mosque, and do not normally confuse the two. But in the Poonkudil Mana, differences between the two kinds of spaces seemed to have been effaced, and patients were sometimes unsure how to behave or what to expect, as our case studies illustrate. The important point is that all three activities—consulting with the patient, prescribing medications, and conducting rituals—were not radically distinguished from each other in terms of their sequence (which varied), place of performance (almost everything was done in the small space where the healers sat), or social/ethnic background of the patient (Hindus, Muslims, and Christians). This mixing of ritual and medicine is perhaps most clearly evident in the healers' annual temple festival, where they worship their lineage deity, but also organize a seminar in which psychologists and psychiatrists are invited for discussions with religious and social leaders, and experts on Ayurveda. This is not unusual in Kerala: there is plenty of evidence from elsewhere in the state for such mixing (Tarabout 1999; Smith 2006: 544 ff.). Nor are such mixings of "religious" with "scientific" instruction unusual in Europe and North America, where Christian hospitals display religious iconography, and most hospitals have chapels and other "religious" spaces.

Like the healers, the patients rarely distinguished between "religious" and "material" complaints and causes: physical diseases were sometimes held to have religious causes, and religious problems were sometimes solved with a dose of medication. Most clients carried different "lists" with them; for example medical prescriptions with psychiatrists' diagnoses, astrologers' reference letters with the names of afflicting heavenly agents, and the prescriptions of the healers from Poonkudil Mana, which were an eclectic mix of ritually charged threads, ashes, cosmopolitan medicines, Ayurvedic medicines meant to be purchased at a nearby traditional pharmacy, and Ayurvedic medicines in modern form such as capsules, to be brought from the nearby town.

Why did healers and patients at Poonkudil Mana not respect the separation of religion and science? Such a question betrays an implicit modernist bias, because it assumes that such a separation is logical and natural, the default position of rational medicine once the layers of culture (e.g., religious belief) have been stripped away. It reflects what Charles Taylor (1993) calls an "acultural" theory of modernity. But why should we assume this? Why should "religious" and "scientific" therapies not be mixed?

The issue is complex. As we emphasized at the beginning of this chapter, modernization theory rests on a sharp distinction between "religion" and "science," and this distinction is particularly strong in cosmopolitan medicine and psychiatry, which systematically attempt to remove any vestige of religion and ritual from their therapies (Sax 2010). We argued that recent developments in what one might call "government-sponsored Ayurveda" in India have followed this model, and this is confirmed by Halliburton's *Mudpacks and Prozac* (2009), which describes practices at a nearby government Ayurveda mental hospital. These are thoroughly nonritualistic and secular, as indeed are the practices at most government Ayurvedic clinics, who thereby contribute to what Latour calls the work of "purification."

And yet the persistence of religious and ritual therapies outside of the medical establishment shows that, for patients at least, they still constitute important therapeutic resources. As Davar and Lohokare show in their chapter (this volume), religious and ritual therapies are quite common in India, and the Poonkudil Mana provides one example. And they are common elsewhere as well. A quick glance through the medical and psychiatric journals suggests that around a quarter of psychiatric patients in the United States use prayer and other religious techniques to deal with their problems; the figure for prayer (and exorcism!) jumps to 30 percent in Switzerland.[19] Nevertheless, mainstream psychiatry, as a branch of "modern" medicine, is reluctant to incorporate into its methods anything that smacks of "religion" (Fallot 1998; Sloan et al. 2000; Kaiser 2007; Koenig 2008; Mueller et al. 2001).

From Latour's perspective, no one has ever been modern, because the ideology on which the notion of "modernity" is based (a strict separation of nature from culture, and hence of science from religion) is untenable. Nature and culture are part of the same world: the natural environment is continually made and remade by humans, while *homo sapiens* makes himself "human" by appropriating natural objects. Medicine, whether ritual, Ayurvedic, or cosmopolitan, is a human activity whose ever-changing theories and practices are in large part determined by culture and history. That is why modernist "purifiers" who insist on separating nature from culture, or science from religion, are fighting a losing battle, since the distinction they wish to preserve is ideological, not ontological. The continuing relevance of religious and ritual therapies, in Europe and North America as well as in India, suggests that medicine and psychiatry will never be "purified" of such practices. Perhaps they should not be.

Notes

1. Weber meant many different things by "rationalization," including the disenchantment of the world, intellectualization, sublimation through knowledge, control of "natural drives," ethical rationalization, democratization, depersonalization (of power, for example), universalization, systematization (of ethics, legal norms, etc.) according to particular principles (Weiss 1981: 48). In general, however, and particularly in relation to the argument we seek to develop here, one can say that for Weber, rationalization refers to the systematization of personal conduct as well as institutional forms, in relation to some overarching norm or principle (e.g., the separation of religion from science; see below).

2. E.g., Lerner 1958, Rogers 1962, and Rostow 1960.

3. Leslie attributed this term to Fred Dunn, who taught at the University of California at San Francisco.

4. See Sax 2009, Chapter VIII, "Postcript: Ritual Healing and Modernity."

5. This distinction was the animating idea of a two-year interdisciplinary research project that supported Sax's research and led to this article, funded by the German Research Council and involving anthropologists, historians, and psychologists, entitled *Asymmetrical Translations: Mind and Body in European and Indian Medicine*. The project was part of the Cluster of Excellence "Asia and Europe in a Global Context" and was followed by an even larger interdisciplinary project entitled "Changing Minds." For more information, see http://www.asia-europe.uni-heidelberg.de/en/home.htm

6. This charismatic healer is described in Smith (2010), and Tarabout (1999).

7. Cf. Tarabout 1999: 140, reporting that the healers' attitude toward psychology was "rather negative."

8. Cf. Sax's discussion of the important West Himalayan demon Masan: much to his surprise, Sax realized only after several years of fieldwork that Masan is multiple and not single (2009).

9. During the *āratī* ritual an illuminated lamp is waved in front of the face of a guest, or a god, to show him or her respect.

10. This red liquid, called *guruti*, is made by mixing slaked lime and turmeric powder with water. It is symbolically equivalent to blood, and is used in rituals that formerly required animal sacrifice.

11. *Annaprāśana* is the "first feeding of grain" to an infant; one of the classical *saṃskāras* or life-cycle rituals of Hinduism.

12. This is colored powder used to make a floral painting for an annual goddess ritual. It is later distributed and daubed on the forehead, arms, and joints.

13. It is clear from the way she says this that she suspects someone has used sorcery against her.

14. Madhav used a great many English words, which are italicized in the translation.

15. *Kuttichathan* is a local spirit who resembles a small boy. There was a film called "My dear Kuttichathan" in Malayalam, and children's comic books

about him are also available. Chathan Kutti was perhaps Ayesha's alternative name for this possessing spirit.

16. One sovereign equals eight grams, so this gold was worth a great deal of money!

17. Long-term patients were previously chained at Poonkudil Mana, but this is no longer practiced.

18. The only exceptions during Bhaskar's five months' research were a Muslim man who refused a ritual for his sister, and an elderly Hindu woman who refused to take medicines, saying that she had come only for the rituals. On both occasions healers displayed their famous tolerance by calmly dispensing what was demanded.

19. In the early 1990s, more than 30 percent of 343 patients interviewed in Switzerland used ritual prayers and exorcism to counteract their diagnosed psychiatric problems (Pfeifer 1994); a similar study in the United States in the 1990s came up with a figure of 25 percent (Eisenberg et al. 1993); other studies show a very high incidence of using religion for "coping" with mental illness (Koenig et al. 1992; Kirov et al. 1998; Tepper et al. 2001). A study published in Lancet showed that "79 percent of the respondents believed that spiritual faith can help people recover from disease" (Sloan et al. 1999: 353, quoting from T. McNichol. The New Faith in Medicine. *USA Today*. April 7, 1996, 4). In another study of 157 hospitalized adults with moderate to high levels of pain, prayer was second only to pain medications (76 percent versus 82 percent) as the most common self-reported means of controlling pain (Mueller et al. 2001).

References

Eisenberg, David M., Ronald C. Kessler, Cindy Foster, Frances E. Norlock, David R. Calkins, and Thomas L. Delbanco. 1993. "Unconventional Medicine in the United States: Prevalence, Costs, and Patterns of Use." *New English Journal of Medicine* 328: 246–252.

Fallot, Roger D. 1998. "The Place of Spirituality and Religion in Mental Health Services." *New Direction for Mental Health Services* 80: 3–12.

Foucault, Michel. 2008. *The Birth of Biopolitics: Lectures at the Collége de France*. New York: Palgrave Macmillan.

Frankenberg, Roland. 1980. "Medical Anthropology and Development: A Theoretical Perspective." *Social Science & Medicine. Part B: Medical Anthropology* 14(4): 197–207.

Halliburton, M., 2009. *Mudpacks and Prozac : Experiencing Ayurvedic, Biomedical, and Religious Healing*, Walnut Creek, C.A.: Left Coast Press.

Janes, Craig R. 2001. "Tibetan Medicine at the Crossroads: Radical Modernity and the Social Organization of Traditional Medicine in the Tibet Autonomous Region, China." In *Healing Power and Modernity: Traditional Medicine, Shamanism, and Science in Asian Societies*, ed. Geoffrey Samuel and Linda Connor. Westport: Bergin and Garvey, 197–221.

Kaiser, Peter. 2007. *Religion in der Psychiatrie: Eine (un)bewusste Verdrängung?* Göttingen: V&R Unipress.

Kirov, George, Roisin Kemp, Kiril Kirov, and Anthony S. David. 1998. "Religious Faith after Psychotic Illness." *Psychopathology* 31: 234–245.

Koenig, Harold G. 2008. "Religion and Mental Health: What Should Psychiatrists Do?" *Psychiatric Bulletin* 32: 201–203.

Koenig, Harold G., Harvey J. Cohen, Dan G. Blazer, Carl Pieper, Keith G. Meador, Frank Shelp, Veeraindar Goli, and Bob DiPasquale. 1992. "Religious Coping and Depression among Elderly, Hospitalized Medically Ill Men." *American Journal of Psychiatry* 149(12): 1693–1700.

Langford, Jean M. 2002. *Fluent Bodies: Ayurvedic Remedies for Postcolonial Imbalance (Body, Commodity, Text)*. Durham: Duke University Press.

Lerner, Daniel. 1958. *The Passing of Traditional Society: Modernizing the Middle East*. Glencoe, I.L.: The Free Press.

Leslie, Charles. 1976a. "Introduction." In *Asian Medical Systems: A Comparative Analysis*, ed. Leslie Charles. Berkeley, Los Angeles, London: University of California Press, 1–12.

———. 1976b. "The Ambiguities of Medical Revivalism in Modern India." In *Asian Medical Systems: A Comparative Analysis*, ed. Leslie Charles. Berkeley, Los Angeles, London: University of California Press, 356–367.

Mueller, Paul S., David J. Plevak, and Teresa A. Rummans. 2001. "Religious Involvement, Spirituality, and Medicine: Implications for Clinical Practice." *Mayo Clinic Proceedings* 76(12): 1225–1235.

Naraindas, Harish. 2006. "Of Spineless Babies and Folic Acid: Evidence and Efficacy in Biomedicine and Ayurvedic Medicine." *Social Science & Medicine* 62(11): 2658–2669.

Nichter, Mark, and Mimi Nichter. 2010. "Revisiting the Concept of Karma: Lessons from a Dhanvantri Homa." *Journal of Ritual Studies* 24(2): 37–55.

Pfeifer, Samuel. 1994. "Belief in Demons and Exorcism in Psychiatric Patients in Switzerland." *British Journal of Medical Psychology* 67(3): 247–258.

Pletsch, Carl E. 1981. "The Three Worlds, or the Division of Social Scientific Labor, circa 1950-1975." *Comparative Studies in Society and History* 23(4): 565–590.

Quack, Johannes, and William S. Sax. 2010. "Introduction: The Efficacy of Rituals." *The Journal of Ritual Studies* 24(1): 5–12.

Rogers, Everett M. 1962. *The Diffusion of Innovations*. Glencoe, I.L.: The Free Press.

Rostow, Walt W. 1960. *The Stages of Economic Growth: A Non-Communist Manifesto*. Cambridge, U.K.: Cambridge University Press.

Sax, William S. 2009. *God of Justice: Ritual Healing and Social Justice in the Central Himalayas*. New York: Oxford University Press.

———. 2010. "Ritual and the Problem of Efficacy." In *The Problem of Ritual Efficacy*, ed. Johannes Quack, William S. Sax, and Jan Weinhold. New York: Oxford University Press, 3–16.

Sloan, Richard P., Emilia Bagiella, and Tia Powell. 1999. "Religion, Spirituality, and Medicine." *Lancet* 353(9153): 664–667.

Sloan, Richard P., Emilia Bagiella, Larry VandeCreek, and Peter Poulos. 2000. "Should Physicians Prescribe Religious Activities." *The New England Journal of Medicine* 342(25): 1913–1916.

Smith, Frederick M. 2006. *The Self Possessed: Deity and Spirit Possession in South Asian Literature.* New York: Columbia University Press.

———. 2010. *The Higher Powers of Man.* Charleston: Nabu Press.

Tambiah, Stanley J. 1989. "Ethnic Conflict in the World Today." *American Ethnologist* 16(2): 335–349.

Tarabout, Gilles. 1999. "'Psycho-Religious Therapy' in Kerala as a Form of Interaction between Local Traditions and (Perceived) Scientific Discourse." In *Managing Distress: Possession and Therapeutic Cults in South Asia,* ed. Marine Carrin. Delhi: Manohar, 133–154.

Tarabout, Gilles, and Daniela Berti. 2009. *Territory, Soil and Society in South Asia.* Delhi: Manohar Publishers and Distributers.

Taylor, Charles. 1993. "Modernity and the Rise of the Public Sphere." In *The Tanner Lectures on Human Values Vol. 14,* ed. Grethe B. Peterson. Salt Lake City: University of Utah Press, 205–260.

Tepper, Leslie, Steven A. Rogers, Esther M. Coleman, and Newton H. Malony. 2001. "The Prevalence of Religious Coping Among Persons With Persistent Mental Illness." *Psychiatric Services* 52: 660–665.

Weiss, Johannes. 1981. "Rationalität als Kommunikabilität. Überlegungen zur Rolle von Rationalitätsunterstellungen in der Soziologie." In *Max Weber und die Rationalisierung Sozialen Handelns,* ed. Walter M. Sprondel and Constans Seyfarth. Stuttgart: Enke, 39–58.

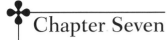

Chapter Seven
Ayurveda in Britain
The Twin Imperatives of Professionalization and Spiritual Seeking

Maya Warrier

Introduction

This chapter examines the role of what is currently the single most important Ayurvedic professional body in the U.K., the Ayurvedic Practitioners Association, to ascertain the effects of professionalization on Ayurveda in Britain. This Association (henceforth "APA") came into being in 2005 in response to the British government's move to introduce statutory regulation of Britain's CAM (Complementary and Alternative Medicine)[1] sector. In the years since its inception, the APA has grown to become the largest and most influential association of Ayurvedic practitioners in Britain. My aim here is to explore the extent to which the APA's efforts to professionalize Ayurveda in response to the government's regulatory initiative has had the effect of "domesticating" this tradition in its British manifestation.

By "domestication" I refer here to the effect that formal systems, institutions, and procedures based on the biomedical model can have on health traditions like Ayurveda, such that the informal, spontaneous, creative, and nonmedicalized networks and lifeworlds upon which it draws for its vitality get restrained and marginalized, if not altogether obliterated.[2] "Domestication" here thus refers to the process whereby creative lifeworlds are "colonized" (in the Habermasian

237

sense) as a result of processes of systematization, standardization, formalization, and institutionalization. The subcultural roots of Ayurveda in the U.K. sustain forms of practice and thinking that lie outside of the regulatory codes and institutional arrangements based largely on the hegemonic biomedical model. When these come to be subsumed by institutionalized frameworks and procedures, the tradition can, through cooptation, lose its capacity to challenge the dominant systems and authority structures put in place by the government. Equally, however, aligning with government policy through the appropriate institutional arrangements guarantees greater protection for the tradition, greater respectability (as a credible and "safe" form of practice) and visibility, as well as greater access to resources (including for instance insurance policies and payments). The success of any organization like the APA lies in its ability to hold its informal networks and formal institutional aspects in creative tension with one another.[3]

To date, the APA has indeed succeeded in retaining its creative lifeworlds and informal networks even while getting increasingly professionalized in accordance with the requirements of statutory regulation. I argue here that rather than institutionalization resulting in the domestication of Ayurveda in Britain, there is some evidence to show that the very opposite has transpired. The regulatory criterion that practitioners of a profession must be organized into one single voluntary body has forced Ayurvedic practitioners from vastly different backgrounds to band together under the APA's wing. The requirement that practitioners go through a process of continuing professional development has meant that they have been forced to share knowledge and skills, and to learn from peers. As a unified interactive professional group, the APA has enabled Ayurvedic member-practitioners in Britain to pool their informal resources, share informal networks and draw upon their creative lifeworlds to an unprecedented degree. The result is a form of professionalized Ayurveda which, though it has a standardized core, branches out from this formalized center to embrace considerable plurality and diversity in worldviews, practices, and modes of therapy and treatment. The result is not domestication but enhanced creativity, heterogeneity, and experimentation.

In all of this, as I will demonstrate here, the APA relies not merely on conceptual and practical ideas intrinsic to Ayurvedic traditions, but more generally on the informal subcultures and lifeworlds of the holistic health (or CAM) sector in the U.K. and beyond. In particular, it relies on this sector's conceptualization of health in terms of the "mind-body-spirit" triad, and draws from the wellsprings of "spirituality" and spiritual seeking that are characteristic of this milieu. Members of the APA are widely networked within the larger holistic health sector and rely on its conceptual and practical resources even as they present a formalized, professionalized face to the British government and the British public.

The findings here draw upon fieldwork conducted among APA members over a period of five years, from 2005, the year of the APA's inception.[4] This chapter relies on in-depth semi-structured interviews with APA members; participant-observation at APA seminars and conferences, Continuing Professional Development (CPD) sessions, and annual retreats, as well as the literature produced by this group in its web pages and periodic newsletters. In what follows, I will first provide a brief overview of Ayurveda in the U.K. and explore the cultural influences that have shaped Ayurveda's development in its British context, before going on to examine the profile and activities of the APA—both its formalized, professionalized aspects, as well as its basis in relatively informal, spontaneous, and creative networks and sources.

Ayurveda in Britain

Ayurveda's key principles and practices no doubt accompanied migrants from the Indian subcontinent whenever they moved in significant numbers to other parts of the world. This would certainly be true of the migration of South Asians to Britain during colonial and postcolonial times. The tradition however tended to remain largely confined to the immigrant groups and seldom spilled out into the larger public domain. It is only since the 1980s that Ayurveda has come to the notice of the larger British (and indeed Western) public. Maharishi Mahesh Yogi's launching of Maharishi Ayurveda in the 1980s provides one of the earliest instances when Ayurveda was promoted and publicized to a Western audience.[5] Since then, Ayurveda has steadily gained in popularity in Britain (and the West generally). The last couple of decades have seen a growing number of British health tourists traveling to India and Sri Lanka to avail themselves of the up-market services offered at Ayurvedic spas, retreats, and hospitals in the subcontinent. Simultaneously, the number of Ayurvedic clinics, treatment centers, and spas in Britain's towns and cities has mushroomed with providers (many of them South Asian immigrants) now publicizing their services through a range of print and electronic media. Following the introduction of U.K.-based training programs in Ayurveda,[6] the number of homegrown therapists and practitioners too has increased significantly. Ayurveda workshops, seminars, and retreats are an increasingly visible feature in Britain's CAM sector. There is a fast-growing list of publications on Ayurveda flooding the print market. Ayurveda has even come to assume brand status, with Indian restaurants in London offering what they call the Ayurvedic *thāli,* and with a range of private companies offering Ayurvedic teas and cosmetics.

Ayurveda entered Britain's public arena at a time when public interest in alternatives to biomedicine was growing. A number of professional organizations working on "holistic health" in the U.K. sprang up in the 1970s and 1980s, some of them securing the patronage of high-profile figures like Prince Charles. The growing demand for alternatives to biomedicine led to a mushrooming of holistic health or CAM traditions in the U.K. CAM traditions, and the holistic health sector, however, have tended to be viewed with considerable suspicion by the British government. As Wujastyk (2005) rightly notes, the government sees CAM systems as something to be tolerated, controlled, regulated and made safe, not because of their potential health benefits but because patients want them. Throughout the opening decade of the new millennium, practitioners of Ayurveda as well as some other CAM traditions in the U.K. have been faced with the prospect of statutory regulation. In the year 2000, a House of Lords Select Committee produced a report that surveyed various aspects relating to the use of Complementary and Alternative Medicine in Britain.[7] In doing so, it divided CAM therapies into three groups, recommending that practices falling into Group 1 be supported. Group 1 included CAM therapies which were increasingly being introduced within the National Health Service; and for which there was some scientific evidence of their real or potential health benefits. Though Ayurveda was initially excluded from Group 1, it came to be included here after intensive lobbying by Ayurveda practitioner groups. This meant that Ayurveda was to be taken seriously, and that it had to submit to the requirements of statutory regulation as proposed in a 2004 Department of Health publication.[8]

The government sought the opinions of Ayurvedic practitioner groups on matters to do with statutory regulation, but it soon became clear that the various groups (more details on these groups to follow later in this chapter) were in complete disagreement with each other. The consultative process ground to a halt. It was at this point that concerned individuals came together to form the Ayurvedic Practitioners Association in an effort to salvage the consultative process and try and secure Ayurveda's interests within the new regulatory framework. APA has had considerable success in bringing the different Ayurvedic practitioner groups together to negotiate with the government. As of October 2013, well over a decade after the publication of the initial House of Lords Select Committee Report in 2000, statutory regulation is yet to be implemented. Moreover, the framework proposed for regulation has been revised and reworked repeatedly by successive governments. The different interest groups to be affected by regulation, who have been gearing up over much of the last decade to meet the regulatory conditions, have for some years now been lobbying the government demanding immediate implementation of the regulatory framework.[9] In the meantime, however, the APA has succeeded in providing Ayurvedic practitioners in the U.K. with a well-organized base from which to lobby the government, and with a relatively secure and professionalized institutional framework within which to practice Ayurveda.

"Medicalized" and "Spiritualized" forms of Ayurveda

The faces and forms of Ayurveda in the U.K. are many and varied. Sifting through all the variety and diversity, however, it is possible to discern two distinct strands of Ayurvedic practice—these are what I refer to here as the "biomedicalized" and the "spiritualized" forms of this tradition. The biomedicalized version has its roots in modern South Asian Ayurvedic practice and owes its presence in Britain to *vaidyas* (Ayurvedic practitioners) who have migrated here in the course of the last half century, and who were previously trained mainly at government colleges of Ayurveda in India and Sri Lanka. These individuals are trained in a version of Ayurveda taught at

South Asian universities and colleges marked by the assimilation of significant aspects of biomedical knowledge into Ayurvedic theory and practice.[10] The curriculum at these institutions, their methods of teaching, and their models of practice all reflect to greater or lesser extents the hegemony of biomedicine in postcolonial India and Sri Lanka. Ayurveda's assimilation of biomedical knowledge and practice in these contexts is evident not just in its formalized training programs but also in its professional associations, its medical journals, and its hospitals, clinics, and pharmaceutical companies. The resultant form of professionalized Ayurveda is a hybrid and pharmaceuticalized system of medicine,[11] offering for the most part health services secondary to, and complementing, those provided by the dominant biomedical system.

The emerging homegrown version of Ayurveda in Britain, while rooted in South Asian forms of biomedicalized Ayurveda, marks a departure from this variant in important respects. It too is a hybrid, and extends beyond both Ayurvedic and biomedical paradigms to embrace the values and practices of Britain's "New Age" milieu of alternative spirituality and holistic health. Even though the majority of individuals teaching on Ayurveda training programs in the U.K. are products of South Asian institutions, their students are for most part not constrained by the form of knowledge and practice they encounter here. They combine what they learn here with paradigms and values derived from the Western holistic health milieu, keeping alive a form of Ayurveda that taps into lifeworlds infused with spiritual seeking and esoteric meaning.[12] The result is Ayurveda in its spiritualized form—an assimilative version of Ayurveda that combines biomedicalized elements derived from South Asia, with orientations and practices central to the loosely defined "mind-body-spirit" framework of Western traditions of holistic health.

My interviews with members of the APA revealed that the vast majority of individuals who had undergone training programs in Ayurveda in the U.K. described themselves as spiritual seekers. Their engagement with Ayurveda formed part of a questing for deeper truths and insights that they believed could be gleaned from ancient traditions like Ayurveda. Many were drawn by the promise of the mystical and esoteric understood to lie at the heart of Ayurveda. Most such individuals are influenced by popular U.S.-based gurus like Deepak Chopra, Vasant Lad, Robert Svoboda, David Frawley, and Maya Tiwari who promote versions of Ayurveda that are heavily infused with modern spirituality.[13] In their own practice, these individuals are concerned to use Ayurveda's principles and practices not merely as a form of remedial medicine, but also, and more importantly, as a means for promoting health through enabling self-knowledge.

This spiritualized version of Ayurveda, which offers interesting points of contrast to the medicalized version, is rooted in the traditions and values of Britain's holistic health milieu. This milieu, as a number of scholars have noted,[14] is marked by certain distinctive characteristics. Unlike in the biomedical sector, the emphasis here is on healing the person rather than curing disease. With its focus not just on physical health, but on the connections among mind, body, and spirit, this sector emphasizes mental and spiritual healing as central to its therapeutic modalities. Spirituality as understood here is closely linked with notions of responsibility, transformation, and empowerment through self-knowledge. Self-knowledge is directly linked to the idea that through the administering of a questionnaire, one's individual *prakṛti* or constitution can be identified in terms of predominant *doṣa(s)*, and that thus identifying one's *doṣa* "type" in turn sheds light on one's entire physical, emotional, and psychological makeup. Promoting health is then about following the generalized lifestyle and dietary regimen prescribed for each *doṣa* type.

Belief in "energy," "energetics," and the "human energy field" are central to the holistic milieu as a whole, and within this milieu, Ayurveda comes to be understood as, among other things, a form of energy healing. Particularly relevant here are Zimmermann's (1992) observations about the "flower power" of modern forms of Ayurveda. The more violent cathartic methods used in traditional Ayurveda, including for instance methods of purgation and emesis, are marginalized here; instead what is emphasized is a form of Ayurveda that is gentle, relaxing, and aesthetically pleasing. The reliance on noninvasive and nonviolent methods is emphasized as a feature that distinguishes Ayurveda from biomedicine.

A major concern for promoters and practitioners of Ayurveda in its spiritualized variant is stress relief. Ayurveda clinics, retreats, and spas are presented as oases of calm in an otherwise rushed world. These sites are often located in areas of scenic beauty; consultations, massages, and other therapy sessions take place in calming interiors

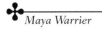

where candles, fragrances, music, and "Vedic" chanting, are all put to good use to create an atmosphere of serenity. In these settings Ayurveda often appears combined with some elementary aspects of modern postural and meditational yoga. Ayurvedic massages take place to the accompaniment of soft, relaxing music, and yoga and meditation sessions are directed at finding a center of stillness within the self. As a tradition now linked with spiritual seeking, Ayurveda in the U.K. thus appears somewhat sacralized. As part of a larger holistic health sector somewhat skeptical of biomedicine and its methods, Ayurveda in the U.K. also offers an implicit critique of the biomedical model, a point I will take up in greater detail later in this chapter.

Professionalizing Ayurveda in Britain: The Ayurvedic Practitioners Association

In 2000 when the government first introduced its regulatory initiative, there were three professional associations operating in the field of Ayurveda in Britain. The first was the Maharishi Ayurvedic Practitioners Association (MAPA), comprising mainly qualified medical doctors practicing Maharishi Ayurveda. The second was the British Association of Accredited Ayurvedic Practitioners (BAAAP) set up in 1999 and allied with a commercial organization, the Ayurvedic Company of Great Britain (ACGB). The founding members of BAAAP were primarily qualified practitioners of Indian origin. Though the parent concern, ACGB, and its many allied organizations, were declared insolvent and closed down in 2008, BAAAP continues to operate with a very small membership.[15] It is noteworthy that until its closure, ACGB ran an Ayurveda undergraduate degree program in London, initially validated by London's Thames Valley University and subsequently offered in association with the Manipal Academy of Higher Education (Mangalore, South India). The third practitioners' association was the Ayurvedic Medical Association (AMA), which came into being in 1996. This was a professional association of qualified Indian and Sri Lankan Ayurvedic practitioners. For a time this group offered Ayurvedic training at the College of Ayurveda U.K. in Milton Keynes. In 2005, the AMA sought formal university accreditation for its course from Middlesex University in London and has, since then, run degree programs at the University's Archway Campus in north London.

Following the government initiative to introduce statutory regulation of Ayurveda, one of the biggest problems facing the different groups representing this tradition was their failure to agree on standardized processes and procedures, particularly in relation to the education and training of aspiring practitioners. ACGB (and the allied practitioners' association, BAAAP) in particular, was openly antagonistic to the other groups involved in the discussions, seeing itself as the only group promoting "authentic" Ayurveda. Much of this objection rested on the question of who was officially "qualified" to serve as a spokesperson for Ayurveda in the U.K. In the view of the ACGB, Indians alone could truly speak for Ayurveda; its objections against other groups were based paradoxically *both* on its claims to be a true inheritor (as an Indian venture) of what it described as this "ancient" and "sacred" tradition, *and* on its claims to represent modern, biomedicalized, government-sponsored Indian Ayurveda. ACGB's tirade against "inauthentic" Ayurveda and its so-called "Western dilution" grew increasingly shrill and strident in the years preceding its eventual closure.[16]

It was in this highly fraught atmosphere that individuals from the other practitioner associations, the MAPA and the AMA, together with a handful of graduates who had received Ayurveda training at Thames Valley University, decided to get together in an attempt to break the impasse in the negotiations on statutory self-regulation. In March 2005, they formed the Ayurvedic Practitioners Association. In contrast with ACGB's exclusivist and oppositional strategy (which relied on assertions of its own "authenticity" and credibility in opposition to what it portrayed as the inauthentic "other"), the APA followed an approach that was inclusive, and opened its doors to practitioners from diverse backgrounds. Moreover, in contrast to the Indian chauvinism and anti-West sentiments discernible in ACGB's representations of Ayurveda (as a great and ancient Indian tradition in danger of dilution by a stereotypically "shallow" and "exploitative" West), the APA promoted a cosmopolitan and humanitarian vision which sought to unify rather than divide. This was reflected in its official vision statement: "To facilitate the health, happiness and well-being of all, we manifest the truth of Ayurveda through unity and love."[17]

The Ayurvedic Practitioners Association was set up as a private company limited by guarantee, aiming to promote and monitor the ethical and professional practice of Ayurveda in Britain. Among its stated objectives were: to ensure that Ayurveda is protected as an independent system of medicine under U.K. and EU law; to generate awareness about Ayurveda and its benefits among the public in order to empower people in their health care choices; to maintain a register of accredited practitioners; to afford regular opportunities for their Continuing Professional Development; and to protect the safety and interests of potential clients/patients by ensuring that its members complied with the APA's Code of Ethics and Professional Conduct.[18] In relation to the government and its regulatory initiatives, it aimed to "actively assist the development and implementation of appropriate statutory self regulation for Ayurveda in the UK," and to represent and campaign on behalf of Ayurveda with respect to any current or intended law, statute, or regulation likely to affect the practice of Ayurveda.[19]

On its web pages, the APA describes itself as "a unifying professional association, guided by the principles of inclusion, transparency and accountability."[20] Among the key aspirations of the founding members of the APA, as laid out in its constitution, is that this organization and its members should be recognized by the government, the public, and the health industry as "synonymous with excellence and professionalism." The Ayurveda that the APA valorizes is "safe," contained, professional, and amenable to statutory self-regulation as required by government authorities.

In keeping with this commitment to professionalism and transparency, and unlike the other associations of Ayurvedic practitioners in Britain, which would appear to have been run on a relatively informal basis (often leaving little by way of paper trails), the APA is structured along formal lines; its policies and procedures, as well as the scope and range of its activities, are clearly documented and readily accessible on its comprehensive and user-friendly website. Through the tireless efforts of its Executive Committee members over the first five years since its inception, the APA succeeded to some extent in winning for itself, and for Ayurveda, formal recognition from the government and from other health professionals in Britain's CAM sector. The APA's commitment to a unifying and inclusive approach has played a significant role in enabling this success. From the start, the APA enjoyed cordial relations with two of the other Ayurvedic practitioner associations—the Maharishi Ayurvedic Practitioners Association (MAPA), as well as the Ayurvedic Medical Association (AMA)—and actively cooperated with these to try and protect the interests of Ayurvedic practitioners in the U.K.[21] In 2007, the three practitioners associations, the AMA, MAPA, and APA, decided to come together to create a unified U.K. register of Ayurvedic practitioners in order to comply with the regulatory criterion that practitioners of a profession must be organized into one single voluntary body.

Though the APA's office bearers were treated with unrelenting hostility by the ACGB in the early years of its operations, this did not deter them from inviting the practitioner association allied with the ACGB, the BAAAP, to open dialogue on the matter of statutory regulation. Over time the APA took on board many of the concerns expressed by BAAAP (and ACGB) regarding the maintenance of high standards of Ayurvedic training and practice in the U.K., and worked hard at negotiating with the government on these matters. BAAAP, however, chose not to merge its register with that of the APA, preferring to continue as "a completely independent organisation to protect the authenticity of Ayurvedic knowledge."[22] Collaboration between the (then) BAAAP President and APA executives led to the development of a peer-reviewed Ayurveda curriculum for U.K. trainees, which was approved by the government of India. This approved Ayurvedic curriculum at graduate and postgraduate levels in the U.K. is closely modeled on the biomedicalized Ayurveda curriculum at Indian institutions.

Along with its allies in the U.K., the APA has worked toward securing agreement on the professional titles for qualified Ayurveda professionals (as "Ayurvedic practitioner" and "Ayurvedic therapist"). It has in place a mandatory Continuing Professional Development (CPD) policy for members and runs a range of CPD seminars and workshops throughout the year led by its own members as well as experts from South Asia, the United States, and Europe. It runs an Approved Supplier Scheme that facilitates quality control of Ayurvedic products used by its members. It also runs a New Members Scheme that allows newly qualified practitioners a year's mentoring from more experienced and established members. These are all measures deemed necessary within the proposed regulatory framework.

The APA sought cordial relations with the other big players in the CAM sector involved in the negotiations leading up to statutory self-regulation. It sought and gained membership of the European

Herbal Practitioners Association (EHPA),[23] which had been designated by the Department of Health as the lead organization for developing draft guidelines required for the regulation of herbal and traditional medicine practitioners.[24] By establishing good working relations with EHPA, the APA was able to actively consult with other CAM professionals, stakeholders, and regulation partners, raise the profile of Ayurveda in this sector, and influence deliberations relating to statutory regulation. The APA's collaborative impulse has led also to the formation and consolidation of international networks of Ayurvedic practitioner groups. It is signed up to international cooperation agreements with counterparts in the United States and Europe.

In all of this, the APA has been something of a model professional association in terms of its cooperative and considered engagement not just with the government and its regulatory initiatives, but also with its partners in the CAM sector, and with the body of Ayurveda practitioners it represents. This has been enabled not least by the presence of articulate, efficient, and dedicated personnel among its founder-members and office bearers, who in turn possess multiple cultural competencies, and skills in organization, diplomacy, networking, and public relations. Since regulation, in its turn, confers a certain degree of respectability, recognition, and credibility upon the traditions regulated,[25] it is no surprise that most Ayurvedic practitioners and groups in Britain have tended not only to welcome the regulatory initiative, but also to rally around the APA in its efforts to standardize and unify Ayurvedic practice in accordance with the proposed regulatory framework. As noted earlier, however, after years of gearing up for statutory self-regulation, groups like the APA are now faced with the prospect of having to contend with a somewhat different regulatory framework than the one they had been led to expect by the previous (Labour) government. This may mean a significant rethinking of their own role and activities as an umbrella organization for Ayurvedic practitioners in the U.K.[26]

Eluding Domestication: The Alternative Lifeworlds of the Holistic Health Sector

The APA's attempts to professionalize and standardize Ayurveda in the U.K. could have resulted in the domestication and impoverishment of this tradition. My field-based research on the APA to date suggests, however, that this has not been the case so far. Ayurveda, as promoted and practiced by those allied with the Ayurvedic Practitioners Association, remains connected with the creative lifeworlds in the holistic health milieu that feed into, nourish, and revitalize this tradition in its British context. Alongside any tendencies toward domestication and standardization one can also discern the opposite—trends toward nurturing and developing a robust informal, creative, and heterogeneous resource-base by drawing upon the "spirituality" that lies at the core of the holistic health network. It is this aspect of the development of Ayurveda in Britain that I will examine in this section.

My findings, based on participant-observation among, and interviews with, APA members over a five-year period (2005–2010), suggest that the Ayurvedic Practitioners Association is best understood as a nodal institution operating within a vast informal network connecting up a range of sociocultural traditions, holistic health therapies, guru-led organizations, networks centering on different forms of popular psychology, meditation groups, and green activism. Members of this Association bring their multiple affiliations, interests, and worldviews to bear on the version of Ayurveda they promote or practice. Since these members come from a great diversity of national and regional backgrounds (including for instance European, North American, South Asian, and Australian), they often feed networks and contacts from these different geographical and cultural locations into the nodal institution. Ideas, symbols, and meanings from different cultures and traditions come together in new and interesting ways often finding novel expression in books authored by these individuals or at workshops, seminars, and retreats led by them. Among them are for instance, individuals qualified in, or at the very least dabbling with, other therapeutic systems like Western herbalism, aromatherapy, spiritual healing, and acupuncture, as well as those with an interest in forms of astrology and *vāstuśāstra*. They include a number of individuals practicing and often teaching different forms of yoga—ranging for instance from the Iyengar method to Bikram yoga. They also include members who take a keen interest in different forms of meditation, often incorporating traditions like *vipassana* and transcendental meditation in their personal practice. A number are affiliated with transnational guru organizations and owe their allegiance to one or more guru.[27] In newsletters, AGM meetings, and CPD sessions, APA members assert a strong commitment to fair trade, conservation, and sustainability in herb production. All these multiple and varied networks and ideologies feed into, and sustain, the APA in its capacity as a nodal institution bringing together a range of worldviews, practices, and paradigms from different sources.

The approach to healing traditions within this network is inclusivist—so that even though healers may choose to specialize in one tradition, they are open to borrowing from other traditions. A therapist specializing in Ayurvedic massage may, for instance, use aspects of aromatherapy or meditation in his or her practice. Similarly an Ayurvedic practitioner qualified in Western herbalism may combine Western herbal remedies with an Ayurvedic understanding of the body's metabolic processes.[28] This inclusivist and integrative approach is very much in evidence in the ethos of the APA—seminars and workshops organized by the APA are very often opportunities for practitioners to learn how elements from other traditions may be used selectively in their own practice.

In some ways, the APA and its members can be understood to constitute a moral community that valorizes an integrative and holistic approach to healing, and prioritizes values such as nurturance and caring; self-understanding, self-awareness, and self-responsibility; as well as experimentation, creativity, and freedom in healing approaches. Subscribers to this worldview are critical of social rules, conventions, roles, and expectations that smother self-expression and self-exploration. A number of the APA's CPD sessions that I attended as participant-observer focused on the importance of the values of caring and nurturance, and on the need for practitioners to be "grounded," unhurried, and empathetic in their dealings with patients. Healers within this moral framework seek the optimization of health—not just in physical but also in emotional, social, and spiritual terms—by enhancing self-awareness and self-understanding on the part of the patient/client. The ideal-typical healer, as portrayed in the APA's CPD sessions, is a calm, sensitive, and caring individual; he or she is creative, self-aware, and patient. He or she possesses good listening skills and is receptive to patients' narratives, allowing for unfettered self-expression on the part of the patient (which is itself understood to be a part of the healing process, leading to greater self awareness and potential self-transformation).

Evident in a number of CPD sessions is an implicit critique of modern lifestyles that afford no time to stop and relax; stress, and the state of being "out-of-touch" with oneself, and out-of-sync with nature and its rhythms, are seen as the root causes of illness in modern Western societies. These features, described in terms of the Ayurvedic *doṣa* triad, are understood to be symptomatic of societies with an excess of *vāta-doṣa*, such that they find themselves constantly in flux and spiraling out of control. What tends to be idealized here is (what is understood to be) a *kapha*-predominant way of life that is calming, stable, "grounded," close to nature, and unhurried.[29] This moral community also devalues authoritarianism in any form and emphasizes a democratic and participatory approach not just to healing but also to all forms of decision making both within its own institutional confines and beyond.

Attitudes toward biomedicine are shaped by this moral and ethical framework. Even though APA members tend to be open to the use of biomedical methods where necessary, they are for most part critical of biomedicine's exclusive preoccupation with treating disease, of its understanding of disease in purely somatic terms, and of its excessive reliance on drugs and invasive medical procedures to combat disease. They are critical also of biomedicine's tendency to generate and sustain significant power imbalances between practitioner and patient. In practical and ideological terms, the integrationism central to attitudes and worldviews in the holistic health sector is very much in evidence in the way APA members engage with biomedicine. Though the biomedical paradigm is viewed with some skepticism, it is valued for its signal contribution to fighting disease, and its tools and methods are selectively appropriated for healing purposes. Biomedicine is understood to yield benefits, but only within its narrow (somaticized) definitions of health and disease. Ayurveda is understood to be broader in scope by virtue of its nonreductionist and "holistic" appreciation of health in somato-psycho-spiritual terms. Ironically, from this perspective, it is not Ayurveda that serves as an adjunct to biomedicine but biomedicine that occupies a subsidiary position vis-à-vis Ayurveda. This view, widely held by APA members, finds expression most commonly in their rather dubious claim that Ayurveda, by virtue of its antiquity and its Vedic (revelatory) roots, is the "mother" of *all* (biomedical and other) health traditions and paradigms in the world.

The APA's Continuing Professional Development sessions, which it organizes for its members a number of times each year in keeping with the requirements of statutory regulation, are important occasions where these different ideas, and the practical healing approaches and techniques that they foster, are shared. Members come together as a group, receive updates on regulatory and other developments relating to Ayurveda, and revitalize their sense of community and solidarity. New members get acquainted with their peers and are socialized into the APA's value system. Those running CPD events and workshops range from the APA's own members to invited guests from different parts of the world, and have included such well-known figures in transnational Ayurveda circles as Vasant Lad, Robert Svoboda, David Frawley, Atreya Smith, and Claudia Welch. A range of *vaidyas* from South Asia have on different occasions led workshops and seminars offering advice on the Ayurvedic treatment of particular conditions. CPD sessions are usually preceded, and often followed, by *pūjās*, the chanting of Sanskrit *ślokas*, and in some cases, the singing of *kīrtan* and *bhajans*. In keeping with the Ayurvedic emphasis on healthy eating, home-cooked food is often served at mealtimes when the CPD sessions take place, and the atmosphere is invariably relaxed, friendly, and welcoming. The sessions tend to be interactive, promoting audience participation, and considerable emphasis is placed on the sharing of good practice, relating especially to practitioner-client interactions. These are also important social events where friends and acquaintances exchange news and gossip, and update each other on events and publications of mutual interest and relevance. These events tend to be unhurried and relaxed, and are often conceptualized as islands of calm that afford a pause from pressured living.

The CPD sessions focusing on Ayurveda and its treatment modalities can broadly be classified into three types. The first type of CPD session focuses on Ayurveda as a system of remedial medicine. Experienced practitioners demonstrate the processes of diagnosis and prescription by examining patients with specific complaints (mainly through a question-answer routine) before an assembled audience and discuss their condition in some depth. In some cases, practitioners lecture on the ways in which Ayurvedic remedies can be used to treat particular (mostly chronic) conditions like psoriasis, eczema, arthritis, obesity, and migraine. In this type of session the focus is very much on the physical manifestations of disease and their treatment.

The second type of CPD session locates Ayurveda within what is understood to be the larger "Vedic" corpus—a body of knowledge believed to contain all manner of ancient esoteric insights from the Indian subcontinent. These sessions are concerned to recover what are understood to be the "Vedic" truths relating to yoga and *prānāyāma, jyotiṣ* (astrology), gemology, and *vāstusāstra,* and to harness these traditions for health promotion, disease prevention, as well as for therapeutic and healing purposes. Many of the more well-known practitioners and promoters of Ayurveda in the West, including for instance the late Maharishi Mahesh Yogi, as well as Vasant Lad, David Frawley, and Robert Svoboda, emphasize Ayurveda's links with these other "Vedic" systems and present somewhat simplified versions of these traditions either for use in Ayurvedic clinical settings or for incorporation into everyday routines and life-style patterns.

The third type of CPD session engages with Ayurveda·as a system of psychosomatic healing. Central to the worldview of the APA and its members, as noted earlier, is the perception of health, healing, and disease not just in physical, but also emotional, psychological, and sociomoral terms. Some APA members go so far as to view psychological stress, imbalances/blockages of the mind, and a lack of self-awareness as the root cause of all disease. Health-seeking and health-optimizing behavior, as understood within this framework, is inseparable from what is understood to be the all-important quest for self-knowledge ("spirituality") and a healthy mind. This mind-body approach to health, promoted most notably by the popular writer and healer Deepak Chopra, is reflected in many of the CPD events hosted by the APA, including, for instance, sessions on "Ayurvedic Psychology: the Healing of Consciousness";[30] "Spirituality in Practice";[31] "Mind Balancing: Western Psychology and Vedic Wisdom in Practice";[32] and "Self Knowing as the Foundation of Life."[33] The emphasis on "spirituality," psychosomatic healing, and "Vedic truth" in the APA, and the readiness to engage not only with esoteric forms of knowledge but also with rituals like *pūjā* and the chanting of *mantras,* suggests an approach that runs counter to the biomedicalization and rationalization that professionalized Ayurveda has undergone in its South Asian context. The result, however, is certainly not a return

253

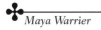

to, or revival of, Ayurveda in its precolonial South Asian form, but the development of an entirely new version of Ayurveda closely wedded to the imperatives of alternative spirituality and holistic health in late-modern Western contexts.

Concluding Remarks

I have argued here that notwithstanding the potential for the domestication of Ayurveda in Britain as a result of the government's regulatory initiative, developments thus far suggest that any such effort to constrain, contain, and standardize Ayurvedic practice will be restricted in scope. Ayurveda practitioners in Britain, and the leading professional organization representing the interests of the Ayurvedic community, have welcomed and willingly embraced regulatory measures intended to professionalize and standardize Ayurvedic practice, in order to ensure its safety and accountability. Rather than submit completely to institutionalized systems, however, the APA has succeeded to date in straddling a middle ground between the regulatory constraints of the mainstream, and the creative freedom of the fringe, by holding its formal institutional aspects and its informal networks in creative tension with each other.

The APA's informal networks are firmly entrenched in the larger holistic health milieu in the U.K., and draw deeply from its anti-authoritarian, spiritualized, and pluralistic worldviews and attitudes. The professionalizing efforts of the APA have to some extent had an enabling and empowering effect on this anti-authoritarian subculture; as a nodal institution in the holistic health milieu, the APA has had the effect of pooling its creative resources, connecting together its informal networks, and enabling the sharing of knowledge between its diverse strands. Central to the discourse within this milieu is the focus on "spirituality," which, as I have argued here, plays a significant role in shaping the development of Ayurveda in its British context. "Spirituality" is a crucial means by which the APA and its members mediate the relationship between Ayurveda and biomedicine, often in novel and creative ways. This focus on "spirituality" enables the APA and its members to resist the dominant biomedical paradigm, and to nurture and sustain counterhegemonic and pluralistic forms of Ayurveda in the U.K., which mark a significant departure from the mainstream professionalized version prevalent in the contemporary South Asian context.

Notes

1. Most scholars writing about this sector today critique the label "Complementary and Alternative Medicine" not only because it fails to do justice to the immense diversity characterizing this sector but also because it reflects the hegemonic status of biomedicine, in relation to which all other health traditions are described. In this chapter, I retain this label mainly because it is still in use in policy and consultative documents generated by the British government. Its use accurately reflects the prevalent attitude towards, as well as political marginality of, this sector in contemporary Britain.

2. I have borrowed this term from Fadlon's work, where she defines domestication as the process in which the foreign is rendered familiar and palatable to local tastes (Fadlon 2005: 2). I use the term here in a more narrow sense, as explained above.

3. See Schneirov and Geczic (1996, 2002) and Fadlon (2005) for comparable studies on the tensions resulting from the formalization and institutionalization of the holistic health sector in the United States and Israel respectively. Reddy (2000) provides an insightful overview of the "professionalising dilemma" facing Ayurveda practitioners in the United States as to whether to emphasize the "religious" aspect of their activities or to present themselves as practicing "medicine."

4. The fieldwork for this project was funded by a Wellcome Trust History of Medicine Project Grant (2005–2010).

5. See, for instance, the contributions of Humes, Jeannotat, and Newcombe in Wujastyk and Smith, eds., 2008.

6. Currently, Middlesex University, London, offers degree courses in Ayurveda at both undergraduate and postgraduate levels. Until recently, degree courses were offered also by another London-based institution, the Ayurvedic University of Europe, affiliated with Manipal University in South India.

7. *House of Lords Select Committee on Science and Technology's Report on Complementary and Alternative Medicine.* HMSO 2000.

8. *Regulation of Herbal Medicine and Acupuncture. Proposal for Statutory Regulation.* March 2004. Available at http://www.dh.gov.uk/en/Publicationsandstatistics/Publications/PublicationsLegislation/DH_4075447. Accessed 16 February 2010.

9. Delays in implementing regulation have been highly detrimental to this sector. In April 2011, the highly restrictive European Traditional and Herbal Medicines Directive came into effect, curtailing individuals' rights to access (and prescribe) prepared medicines from suppliers and manufacturers. See Frankincense (European Herbal and Traditional Medicine Practitioners Association's Newsletter) January 2010. The regulatory framework,

as currently envisioned, is intended to allow the necessary access to those suitably qualified as "practitioners," but the delay in implementation has meant that practitioners remain highly constrained in their practice.

10. On professionalized Ayurveda's assimilation of biomedicine in South Asia, see Brass 1972; Leslie 1973, 1974, 1976; Langford 2002.

11. See Banerjee 2008, 2009 and Bode 2008 for insights into the process and impact of Ayurveda's pharmaceuticalization in South Asia and beyond.

12. See Warrier 2009, 2011.

13. Comparable studies of spiritualized Ayurveda in the West include Zysk 2001; Reddy 2000, 2002, 2004; Welch 2008.

14. See for instance Beckford 1984, 1985; Heelas 1996, 2008; Bowman 1999, 2000; Hedges and Beckford 2000; Heelas, Woodhead et al. 2004; Partridge 2004–2005.

15. See http://www.britayurpractitioners.com/. Accessed 9 April 2010.

16. An ACGB conference organized on 17 January 2003 on the topic "The Dangers of Western Dilution of Ayurveda" saw a range of speakers from ACGB and its allied organizations, as well as invited speakers from India, lashing out against Western Ayurveda practitioners and warning against the dangers of "diluting" the standards of Ayurveda practice. The 2003 conference was followed by a second one on 4 May 2005 when similar alarmist and anti-West sentiments were expressed by speakers closely allied with the ACGB. The ACGB, which had crucial commercial interests at stake in all of this, claimed sole legitimacy as a body of spokespersons for Ayurveda in Britain. Much of its tirade against "Western Ayurveda" appeared to rely on Indian nationalistic sentiment and exclusivism.

17. See www.apa.uk.com. Accessed 6 April 2010.

18. http://www.apa.uk.com/includes/uploads/file/2010/APA percent20Constitution.pdf. Accessed 6 April 2010.

19. Ibid.

20. www.apa.uk.com. Accessed 6 April 2010.

21. Among the founding members of the APA were members of the AMA and MAPA; the two individuals to have consecutively held the office of APA president to date are both senior Maharishi Ayurveda practitioners.

22. APA News Update—August, September and October 2007. Available at www.apa.uk.com. Accessed 16 February 2010.

23. The APA prompted a name change of EHPA to the more inclusive EHTPA ("T" standing for "Traditional Medicine") in May 2007 to reflect that fact that many of its members, including for instance practitioners of traditional Tibetan medicine and traditional Chinese medicine, besides Ayurveda practitioners, used more than just herbal remedies.

24. Among the members of the EHPA were such professional associations as the Association of Master Herbalists, the British Association of Traditional Tibetan Medicine, the National Institute of Medical Herbalists, and the Register of Chinese Herbal Medicine.

25. See Saks 2002.

26. Current government proposals suggest, for instance, that a centralized body, the Health Professions Council, will, in due course, be charged with maintaining a statutory register of practitioners of traditional and herbal medicines. This body will deal with public complaints, execute disciplinary procedures, and monitor practitioner compliance with CPD requirements and standards of ethical and professional conduct. Tradition-specific associations like the APA will therefore be relieved of this responsibility. See APA News Update—Spring 2011, available at www.apa.uk.com. Accessed 26 November 2011.
27. This information is derived from in-depth personal interviews with members conducted between 2005 and 2010.
28. As in note 27 above. Additionally, websites maintained by individual practitioners, as well as books authored by some of them, indicate the ways in which such combinations are deployed in everyday practice.
29. The qualities associated with *vāta* (understood as a combination of the air and ether elements) are constant activity, transformation, and movement. Those associated with *kapha* (understood as a combination of the elements water and earth) are understood to be conducive to stability, groundedness, and calmness.
30. Two-day CPD seminar with David Frawley, 4 and 5 November 2006.
31. Workshop conducted by Craig Brown, at the APA's "Third Annual Multi-Track Event," 6 and 7 June 2009.
32. CPD session led by Reinhard Kowalski, 30 September and 1 October 2006.
33. Title of two-day CPD seminar with Vasant Lad, 6 and 7 October 2008.

References

Banerjee, Madhulika. 2008. "Ayurveda in Modern India: Standardization and Pharmaceuticalization." In *Modern and Global Ayurveda: Pluralism and Paradigms,* ed. Dagmar Wujastyk and Frederick M. Smith. New York: State University of New York Press, 201–214.

———. 2009. *Power, Knowledge, Medicine: Ayurvedic Pharmaceuticals at Home and Abroad.* Delhi: Orient Black Swan.

Beckford, James A. 1984. "Holistic Imagery and Ethics in New Religious and Healing Movements." *Social Compass* 31(2-3): 259–272.

———. 1985. "The World Images of New Religious and Healing Movements." In *Sickness and Sectarianism: Exploratory Studies in Medical and Religious Sectarianism,* ed. R. Kennet Jones. Gower: Aldershot, 72–93.

Bode, Maarten. 2008. *Taking Traditional Knowledge to the Market: The Modern Image of the Ayurvedic and Unani Industry, 1980-2000.* Hyderabad: Orient Longman.

Bowman, Marion. 1999. "Healing in the Spiritual Marketplace: Consumers, Courses and Credentialism." *Social Compass* 46(2): 181–189.

———, ed. 2000. *Healing and Religion.* Middlesex, U.K.: Hisarlik Press.

Brass, Paul R. 1972. "The Politics of Ayurvedic Education: A Case Study of Revivalism and Modernization in India." In *Education and Politics in India: Studies in Organization, Society, and Policy*, ed. Susanne Hoeber Rudolph and Lloyd I. Rudolph. Cambridge, M.A.: Harvard University Press, 342–371.

Cant, Sarah, and Ursula Sharma. 1996. "Demarcation and Transformation within Homeopathic Knowledge: A Strategy of Professionalisation." *Social Science and Medicine* 42(4): 579–588.

Chandler, Siobhan. 2008. "The Social Ethic of Religiously Unaffiliated Spirituality." *Religion Compass* 2(10): 1–17.

Fadlon, Judith. 2005. *Negotiating the Holistic Turn: The Domestication of Alternative Medicine*. New York: State University of New York.

Hedges, Ellie, and James A. Beckford. 2000. "Holism, Healing and the New Age." In *Beyond New Age: Exploring Alternative Spirituality*, ed. Steven Sutcliffe and Marion Bowman. Edinburgh: Edinburgh University Press, 169–187.

Heelas, Paul. 1996. *The New Age Movement*. Oxford, U.K.: Blackwell.

———. 2008. *Spiritualities of Life: Romantic Themes and Consumptive Capitalism*. Oxford, U.K.: Blackwell.

Heelas, Paul, Linda Woodhead, Benjamin Seel, and Bronislaw Szerszynski. 2004. *The Spiritual Revolution: Why Religion is Giving Way to Spirituality*. Oxford, U.K.: Wiley Blackwell.

Humes, Cynthia Ann. 2008. "Maharishi Ayur-Veda™: Perfect Health™ through Enlightened Marketing in America." In *Modern and Global Ayurveda: Pluralism and Paradigms*, ed. Dagmar Wujastyk and Frederick M. Smith. New York: State University of New York Press, 309–331.

Jeannotat, Francoise. 2008. "Maharishi Ayur-Ved: A Controversial Model of Global Ayurveda." In *Modern and Global Ayurveda: Pluralism and Paradigms*, ed. Dagmar Wujastyk and Frederick M. Smith. New York: State University of New York Press, 285–307.

Langford, Jean M. 2002. *Fluent Bodies: Ayurvedic Remedies for Postcolonial Imbalance*. Durham, N.C.: Duke University Press.

Leslie, Charles. 1973. "The Professionalizing Ideology of Medical Revivalism." In *Modernization of Occupational Cultures in South Asia*, ed. Milton Singer. Durham, N.C.: Duke University Press, 216–242.

———. 1974. "The Modernization of Asian Medical Systems." In *Rethinking Modernization: Anthropological Perspectives*, ed. John J. Poggie and Robert N. Lynch. Westport, C.T.: Greenwood Press, 69–108.

———. 1976. "The Ambiguities of Medical Revivalism in Modern India." In *Asian Medical Systems: A Comparative Study*, ed. Charles Leslie. Berkeley, Los Angeles, London: University of California Press, 356–367.

Newcombe, Suzanne. 2008. "Ayurvedic Medicine in Britain and the Epistemology of Practising Medicine in 'Good Faith.'" In *Modern and Global Ayurveda: Pluralism and Paradigms*, ed. Dagmar Wujastyk and Frederick M. Smith. New York: State University of New York Press, 257–284.

Partridge, Christopher. 2004–2005. *The Re-Enchantment of the West*, Vols. 1 & 2, London and New York: T&T Clark.

Reddy, Sita. 2000. *Reinventing Medical Traditions: The Professionalization of Ayurveda in Contemporary America*. Unpublished Ph.D. thesis, University of Pennsylvania.

———. 2002. "Asian Medicine in America: The Ayurvedic Case." *Annals of the American Academy of Political and Social Science: Global Perspectives on Complementary and Alternative Medicine* 583 (September): 97–121.

———. 2004. "The Politics and Poetics of 'Magazine Medicine': New Age Ayurveda in the Print Media." In *The Politics of Healing: Histories of Alternative Medicine in Twentieth-Century North America*, ed. Robert D. Johnston. London: Routledge, 207–229.

Saks, Mike. 2002. "Professionalisation, Regulation and Alternative Medicine." In *Regulating the Health Professions*, ed. Judith Allsop and Mike Saks. London, Thousand Oaks, New Delhi: Sage Publications, 148–161.

Schneirov, Matthew, and Jonathan David Geczik. 1996. "A Diagnosis for Our Times: Alternative Health's Submerged Networks and Transformation of Identities." *Sociological Quarterly* 37: 627–644.

———. 2002. "Alternative Health and the Challenges to Institutionalization." *Health* 6(2): 201–220.

Warrier, Maya. 2009. "Seekership, Spirituality and Self-Discovery: Ayurveda Trainees in Britain." *Asian Medicine: Tradition and Modernity* 4: 423–451.

———. 2011. "Revisiting the Easternisation Thesis: The Spiritualisation of Ayurveda in Modern Britain." In *Spirituality in the Modern World*, Volume 3, ed. Paul Heelas. London and New York: Routledge, 299–319.

Welch, Claudia. 2008. "An Overview of the Education and Practice of Global Ayurveda." In *Modern and Global Ayurveda: Pluralism and Paradigms*, ed. Dagmar Wujastyk and Frederick M. Smith. New York: State University of New York Press, 129–138.

Wujastyk, Dominik. 2005. "Regulation of Ayurveda in Great Britain in the Twenty-First Century." *Asian Medicine: Tradition and Modernity* 1(1): 162–184.

———. 2008. "The Evolution of Indian Government Policy on Ayurveda in the Twentieth Century." In *Modern and Global Ayurveda: Pluralism and Paradigms*, ed. Dagmar Wujastyk and Frederick M. Smith. New York: State University of New York Press, 43–76.

Wujastyk, Dagmar, and Frederick M. Smith, eds. 2008. *Modern and Global Ayurveda: Pluralism and Paradigms*. New York: State University of New York Press.

Zimmermann, Francis. 1992. "The Gentle Purge: The Flower Power of Ayurveda." In *Paths to Asian Medical Knowledge*, ed. Charles Leslie and Allan Young. Berkeley: University of California Press, 209–223.

Zysk, K. G. 2001. "New Age Āyurveda, or What Happens to Indian Medicine When It Comes to America." *Traditional South Asian Medicine* 6: 10–26.

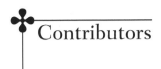

Contributors

Helene Basu is Full Professor of Social Anthropology at Westfaelische Wilhelms-Universitaet Muenster. She has conducted fieldwork in Gujarat on Hindu and Muslim socioreligious practices and identity formations, migration across the Indian Ocean, and the "African diaspora" (Sidi) in Gujarat (ed. *Journeys and Dwellings—Indian Ocean Themes in South Asia,* 2008). Her publications include *Embodying Charisma* (co-edited with Pnina Werbner, 1998) and a book on social memory and Rajput kingship in Kacchch (*Von Barden und Königen. Ethnologische Studien zur Göttin und zum Gedächtnis,* 2004. She is co-editor of the *Encyclopedia of Hinduism* (Brill). Recent research interests concern migration, mental health, and transcultural psychiatry.

Hari Kumar Bhaskaran Nair completed his M.A. in Health and Society in South Asia (MAHASSA) from Heidelberg University in 2010. He was an associate member of the Cluster of Excellence "Asia & Europe" and now works as the Coordinator of NSS group of Ayurveda Hospitals in Kerala, India. His master's thesis, entitled *Marunnum Mantravum: An Ethnographic Enquiry into the Patterns of Affliction and Therapeutics in a Traditional Healing Practice in Malabar, North Kerala,* is published online on Savifa, the Heidelberg University's digital library on South Asian studies.

Laurence J. Kirmayer, M.D., is James McGill Professor and Director of the Division of Social and Transcultural Psychiatry in the Department of Psychiatry, McGill University. He is Editor-in-Chief of the journal *Transcultural Psychiatry.* He directs the Culture & Mental Health Research Unit at the Institute of Community and Family Psychiatry, Jewish General Hospital in Montreal. He founded and directs the annual Summer Program and Advanced Study

Institute in Cultural Psychiatry at McGill. He co-edited the volumes *Current Concepts of Somatization* (American Psychiatric Press), *Understanding Trauma: Integrating Biological, Clinical, and Cultural Perspectives* (Cambridge University Press), and *Healing Traditions: The Mental Health of Aboriginal Peoples in Canada* (University of British Columbia Press), *Cultural Consultation: Encountering the Other in Mental Health Care* (Springer), and *Revisioning Psychiatry: Cultural Phenomenology, Critical Neuroscience and Global Mental Health* (Cambridge). He is a Fellow of the Canadian Academy of Health Sciences.

Harish Naraindas is Associate Professor at the School of Social Sciences, Jawaharlal Nehru University, New Delhi. He is also Adjunct Associate Professor at the University of Iowa and was Joint-Appointments Professor (2008–2012) of the Cluster of Excellence at the South Asia Institute, University of Heidelberg. He has published on a range of topics, including the emergence of tropical medicine as a discipline, the history of smallpox, Ayurveda, and the German Kur, in leading journals such as the *Contributions to Indian Sociology, Indian Economic and Social History Review, Asian Journal of Social Sciences, Social Science & Medicine,* and the *Zeitschrift für Ethnologie.* He has recently co-edited a special issue of *Anthropology and Medicine* (April 2011) on medical tourism.

Johannes Quack earned a Ph.D. in Social Anthropology at Heidelberg University in 2009. He was a postdoctoral fellow at the Cluster of Excellence "Asia & Europe," Heidelberg University and the Division of Social and Transcultural Psychiatry, McGill University, Montreal. Currently he is principal investigator of the Emmy Noether-Project "The Diversity of Nonreligion" at Goethe-University Frankfurt. Quack is the author of *Disenchanting India: Organized Rationalism and Criticism of Religion in India* (OUP, 2012), co-editor of *The Problem of Ritual Efficacy* (OUP, 2010), and co-editor of *Religion und Kritik in der Moderne* (LIT, 2012).

William S. ("Bo") Sax studied at Banaras Hindu University, the University of Wisconsin, the University of Washington (Seattle), and the University of Chicago, where he earned a Ph.D. in Anthropology in 1987. He has taught at Harvard University, the University of

Canterbury in Christchurch, New Zealand, and at Heidelberg University, where he is Chair of Ethnology at the South Asia Institute. His major works include *Mountain Goddess: Gender and Politics in a Central Himalayan Pilgrimage* (1991), *The Gods at Play: Lila in South Asia* (1995), *Dancing the Self: Personhood and Performance in the Pandav Lila of Garhwal* (2002), *God of Justice: Ritual Healing and Social Justice in the Central Himalayas* (2008), and *The Problem of Ritual Efficacy* (2010).

Maya Warrier is Associate Professor in Religious Studies at the University of Wales, Trinity Saint David, U.K. Her research interests center on the construction and transformation of religious identities and traditions in modern transnational contexts with particular reference to contemporary Hinduism. She is author of *Hindu Selves in a Modern World: Guru Faith in the Mata Amritanandamayi Mission* (Routledge-Curzon, 2005) and co-editor of *Public Hinduisms* (Sage, 2012). Her contribution to the current volume is based on a fieldwork-based project, funded by the Wellcome Trust, researching the development of modern forms of Ayurveda in the U.K.

Francis Zimmermann holds the chair of South Asian Anthropology and History of Science at the Ecole des Hautes Etudes en Sciences Sociales (EHESS), Paris. He is the author of several books on Ayurvedic medicine including *The Jungle and the Aroma of Meats: An Ecological Theme in Hindu Medicine*, available at Motilal Banarsidass, Delhi.

✤ Index